Sameen Ali    Peter Anto John
Anthony Chen    John Christy John
Avery Kennedy    Asfar Khan
Arnavi Patel    Nasia Sheikh
April Sui    Belinda Tam
Justine Nicole Banszky    Jeremy Steen
Dr. Austin Mardon

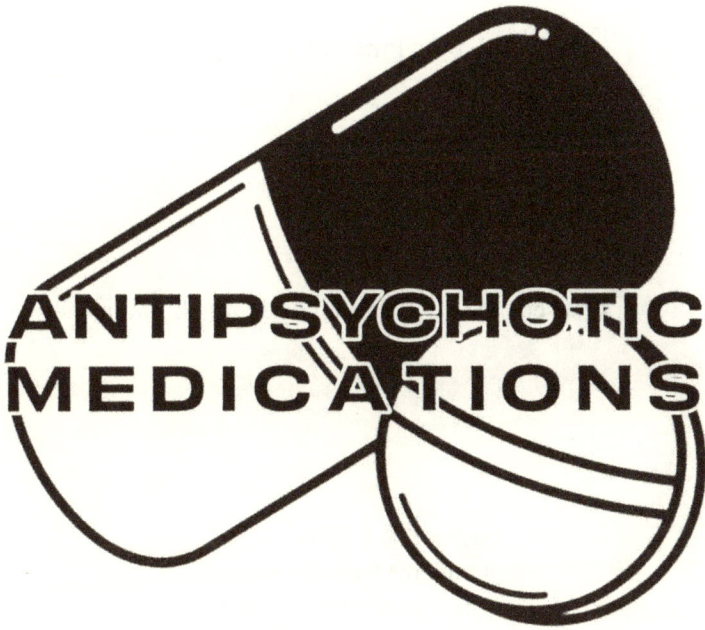

I0071556

# ANTIPSYCHOTIC
# MEDICATIONS

# GM
PRESS

Copyright © 2021 by Austin Mardon
All rights reserved. This book or any portion thereof may not be reproduced
or used in any manner whatsoever without the express written permission
of the publisher except for the use of brief quotations in a book review or
scholarly journal.
First Printing: 2021

Typeset and Cover Design by Jedidiah Emms

ISBN: 978-1-77369-251-7
Golden Meteorite Press
103 11919 82 St NW
Edmonton, AB T5B 2W3
www.goldenmeteoritepress.com

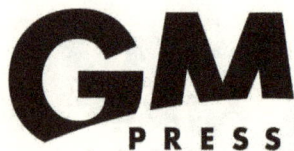

**GM**
PRESS

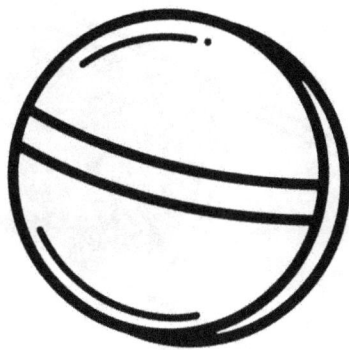

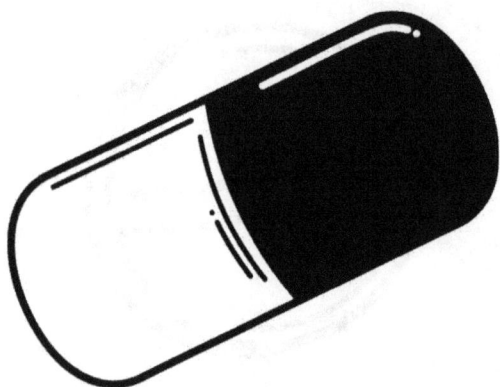

# CONTENTS

# ANTIPSYCHOTIC MEDICATIONS

# CHAPTER 1
## HISTORY, BACKGROUND, AND EARLY USES

### Asfar Khan

Antipsychotics are almost 200 years old and have been discovered serendipitously like many other scientific discoveries. Today, the drug is primarily used medically in the treatment of symptoms like delusions, hallucinations, paranoia or disordered thought associated with psychosis and schizophrenia (1-3). Both negative and positive symptoms are treated for schizophrenic patients through antipsychotic medications. They are also used to treat psychosis that may occur from bipolar disorder, depression, and Alzheimer's disease. They may also be beneficial in regards to stabilizing mood in bipolar disorder, reducing anxiety, as well as reducing tics in other syndromes such as Tourette (1-3). Generally, these medications have sedative effects that can be used to help calm or clear confusion in individuals experiencing acute psychosis. However, it should be noted that these medications do not cure the condition, rather control the symptoms. When taken over a longer duration, antipsychotics can prevent further episodes of psychosis (1).

Antipsychotic medications have generally been classified as typical and atypical antipsychotics (2). The classical antipsychotics include phenothiazines and butyrophenones, while the atypical primarily include benzamides (2). Initially, forms of antipsychotic therapy included electroconvulsive therapy, insulin coma, frontal lobotomy and sedation (1,2). This was until the discovery of chlorpromazine, which was a form of phenothiazine. Chlorpromazine was the first to revolutionize psychiatric practice, and replace these traditional therapies. Phenothiazines had originally been used in the dyeing industry, and for medical treatment such as antiseptics and anthelmintics (1). In this chapter we will discuss the history and development of antipsychotic medications, as well as briefly address the uses and effects of antipsychotics. A more thorough deep dive on the uses, effects, and impacts of antipsychotic medications will be explored in later chapters.

In 1856, William Henry Perkin created a blue dye during an experiment attempting to create quinine from tar (1). This blue dye sparked a rise in the commercial dye industry and led to the creation of methylene blue in 1876 (1,2). Methylene blue was a derivative of phenothiazine and was what led to the discovery of phenothiazine a few years later (1). In 1891, Paul Erlich discovered that methylene blue was effective at treating malaria symptoms (1). Following this, Werner Schulemann and colleagues attempted to uncover and synthesize other compounds related to methylene blue (1). A compound to come out of this discovery was diethylaminomethyl, a derivative of methylene blue (1). This derivative proved to have even more antimalarial properties in comparison to its predecessor methylene blue. However, this was found to be too toxic to have any form of clinical application (1). Later down the line, Schulemann and colleagues discovered quinacrine, which when combined with quinine, served as the primary therapy for malaria globally (1).

In World War II, following the victories of the Japanese, much of the world was denied access to quinine-producing areas of the world, and the search for a synthetic antimalarial agent was on (1,2). This race to discover synthesize an antimalarial agent led to the development of aminoalkyl phenothiazines, however, these did not possess significant antimalarial activity. As things progressed in World War II, Rhone-Poulenc, a French company discovered promethazine (1,2). Promethazine was the first synthetic antihistamine (1). In 1950, H. Laborit, an anesthesiologist, found promethazine to have sedation effects, and that its activity is similar to other anesthetic agents. This led to the rapid application of promethazine in clinical anesthesia.

The widespread application of promethazine as a clinical anesthetic prompted Rhone-Poulenc to search for other phenothiazine derivatives with similar activity. Later in that year, Simone Courvoisier tested chlorpromazine. Chlorpromazine was found to prolong barbiturate-induced sleep in rodents (1). In 1951, Henri Laborit observed that patients sedated by chlorpromazine, promethazine, and other analgesics require lower doses of anesthetic agents (1). They also observed that chlorpromazine led to no loss of consciousness, however did make patients sleepy and uninterested in what was around them (1).

Based on Laborit's observations, chlorpromazine was pushed to be used in clinical applications. Chlorpromazine was supplied to the Central Military

2

and Sainte-Anne Hospital in Paris (1). This was the first reported chlorpromazine treated case. A 57-year-old patient was admitted to the hospital due to erratic and uncontrollable behaviors (2). The patient was noted to have made impassioned political speeches in public cafes and had a record of assaulting strangers (2). After one day of administration of chlorpromazine, the patient was noted to be much calmer (2). After one week, the patient was joking with medical staff, and after three weeks, the patient appeared relatively normal and was discharged (2). Other patients with hyperactive behavior and treated with chlorpromazine showed similar benefits (2).

In 1952, Rhone-Poulenc released chlorpromazine under the name of Largactil, and in 1954 was known as Thorazine (1). This led to the availability of chlorpromazine globally and allowed further trials of the compound. In the late 1950s, the therapeutic effects of chlorpromazine were solidified through the completion of a study by the US Veterans Administration Collaborative Study Group (1). Amongst this, a significant decrease in the prevalence of psychiatric inpatients was witnessed around the world, which was presumably due to the widespread use of chlorpromazine and related drugs.

In 1954, a few years after the release of chlorpromazine for clinical use, side effects such as parkinsonism, dystonia, and akathisia (detailed in later chapters) began to be recognized (1,2). And in 1961, the prevalence of these adverse events were reported in approximately 38.9% of patients who were treated with an antipsychotic drug (1). It was then that clinicians and researchers became aware that there may be a correlation between those adverse events and anti-psychotic drugs. In order to find alternatives to chlorpromazine, German psychiatrists with the help of Wander Pharmaceuticals in Switzerland discovered clozapine (1,2). Clozapine was found to have similar effects to chlorpromazine, however none of the adverse events reported following administration. Following several large clinical trials, clozapine was introduced to European countries in the 1970s (1,2). And in 1973, Gilbert Honigfeld, a clinical psychologist, began an open-label phase 2 trial on prison inmates in the USA (1,2). Clozapine became gradually accepted, showing promising effects as an antipsychotic. However, in 1975, it was found to develop blood dyscrasia in several patients (blood dyscrasia is disease of the blood which may affect the plasma or cellular components of the blood) (2). This inevitably delayed progression of clozapine in the market, however, in 1984 a 6-week double blind study showed clear superiority in clozapine over chlorpromazine (2). Several clinical trials later, clozapine was introduced to the US markets in 1990. Clozapine's initial use in clinics and studies established that it was useful in treating hallucinations, delusions, disorganized behaviour, and disorganized speech associated with schizophrenia (2). Furthermore, it was also used to treat other symptoms such as social withdrawal, and apathy. This led to the creation of atypical antipsychotic drugs in the 90's such as risperidone, olanzapine, quetiapine, ziprasidone, and other similar drugs (1). Although these were considered as effective as the other drugs, they were found to have considerable extrapyramidal side effects (1,2).

### ATYPICAL ANTIPSYCHOTICS

All the atypical antipsychotic medications fall under a group of drugs that are termed mixed receptor antagonists (1). Typical antipsychotics tend to have a three-ring nucleus, however atypical antipsychotic medications do not (1). Atypical antipsychotic medications would include risperidone, olanzapine, and quetiapine. This group of antipsychotics have been found to reduce extrapyramidal syndrome, and treat the negative symptoms of schizophrenia in various double-blind trials (1). Atypical antipsychotics can also be referred to as second generation antipsychotics (SGA), and serotonin-dopamine antagonists (SDA). On the other hand, typical antipsychotics were more likely to cause extrapyramidal side effects, that could affect motor control, cause tremors and spasms, and cause loss of control or muscle movement as discussed below. Currently, there are 7 different types of atypical antipsychotics offered: aripiprazole, clozapine, ziprasidone, paliperidone, risperidone, quetiapine, and olanzapine (3). Ablify (aripiprazole) is used to treat schizophrenia and bipolar disorder (3). Clozaril (clozapine) is used for treatment resistant schizophrenia and suicidal behaviour (3). Geodon (ziprasidone) is used to treat schizophrenia, and manic or mixed episodes of bipolar disorder (3). Invega (paliperidone) is used to treat schizophrenia, and is the only oral atypical antipsychotic. Rispderal (risperidone) is also used to treat schizophrenia, bipolar disorder, and irritability with autism (3). Seroquel (quetiapine) is another atypical antipsychotic used to treat schizophrenia, bipolar, and other mood disorders (3). And finally, Zyprexa (olanzapine) is also used to treat schizophrenia and bipolar disorder) (3).

### USES AND EFFECTS OF ANTIPSYCHOTIC MEDICATIONS

• Sedation: Sedation is a common effect with antipsychotic medications. However, many patients become tolerant to the sedative effect over time. Low dose first generation antipsychotics (FGAs) and clozapine are the most sedating (3).

- Hypotension: Orthostatic hypotension can occur with all antipsychotic medications, predominantly with low-dose FGAs and clozapine. It can also occur with risperidone and quetiapine. This effect is more abundant in older adults, those on blood pressure medications, and those who have other cardiovascular diseases (3).
- Anticholinergic Effects: Anticholinergic effects include constipation, urinary retention, dry mouth, blurred vision and, at times, cognitive impairment. These symptoms can lead to other problems such as tooth decay, falls, or gastrointestinal obstruction (3).
- Extrapyramidal Symptoms: Antipsychotic medications cause four main extrapyramidal symptoms: pseudoparkinsonism, akathisia, acute dystonia, and tardive dyskinesia. Pseudoparkinsonism is a reversible syndrome that results in the shaking of the hands and arms, as well as rigidity or lack of movement in the arms and shoulders. Akathisia is described as a feeling of inner restlessness that can be seen through excessive pacing or inability to remain still for any length of time. Dystonia occurs when there are spastic contractions of the muscles. Tardive dyskinesia is an involuntary movement disorder that can occur with long-term antipsychotic treatment, and may not be reversible even if the medication is discontinued. Abnormal movements from tardive dyskinesia can include myoclonic jerks, tics, chorea, and dystonia (3).
- Hyperprolactinemia: Antipsychotics can increase prolactin levels. Hyperprolactinemia is common with the use of any FGA, as well as with risperidone. Hyperprolactinemia can be asymptomatic, but may cause gynecomastia, galactorrhea, oligo- or amenorrhea, sexual dysfunction, acne, hirsutism, infertility, and loss of bone mineral density. Symptoms often appear within a few weeks of beginning the antipsychotic or increasing the dosage, but can also arise after long-term stable use (3).
- Sexual Dysfunction: Up to 43 percent of patients taking antipsychotic medications report problems with sexual dysfunction, a distressing adverse effect that can lead to poor medication adherence. Use of antipsychotics can affect all phases of sexual function, including libido, arousal, and orgasm. Both FGAs and SGAs can impair arousal and orgasm in men and women. FGAs especially have been found to cause erectile and ejaculatory dysfunction in men (3).
- Agranulocytosis: In rare cases, clozapine may cause neutropenia agranulocytosis that can lead to potentially fatal infections. Risk increases with age, and in females. Because of the risk, the U.S. Food and Drug Administration (FDA) requires that clozapine be available only through programs that monitor white blood cell counts weekly for the first six months, every two weeks for the next six months, and monthly thereafter (3).
- Cardiac Arrhythmias: All antipsychotics can contribute to prolongation of ventricular repolarization which can in turn lead to sudden cardiac death. This effect is most marked with the low-potency FGA thioridazine and the

SGA ziprasidone, and is dose dependent. The incidence of sudden cardiac death among patients taking antipsychotics is about twice that of the general population (3).

• Seizures: All antipsychotics can lower the seizure threshold. They should be used with caution in patients who have a history of seizures and in those with organic brain disorders. Generally, the more sedating the antipsychotic, the more it lowers the seizure threshold. Seizures are most common with low-potency FGAs and clozapine, especially at higher dosages (3).

• Metabolic Syndrome Issues: Weight gain is a common adverse effect of using antipsychotic medications, and can be rapid and difficult to control. Weight gain does not seem to be dose dependent within the normal thera-peutic range. The effect is worse with clozapine and olanzapine; minimal with aripiprazole and ziprasidone; and intermediate with other antipsychot-ics, including low-potency FGAs. Antipsychotic medications can contribute to a wide range of glycemic abnormalities, from mild insulin resistance to diabetic ketoacidosis, as well as worsening of glycemic control in patients with pre-existing diabetes (3).

## TIMELINE OF ANTIPSYCHOTICS

All in all, the history of antipsychotic drug development was initiated with the discovery of chlorpromazine in 1950-1952. Following the discovery of chlorpromazine, majority of the atypical antipsychotic drugs were intro-duced between the later 1950s up until the mid-1970s. Following this era was the widespread use of clozapine, which entered the European markets in the 1970s and the US market in the 1990s. This was the new era of schizo-phrenia and psychosis treatment. By the later 1990s, clozapine, risperidone, olanzapine, and quetiapine (atypical antipsychotics) were available on the US market. The demand of atypical antipsychotics during this time was a re-sult of similar efficacy in treating positive symptoms of schizophrenia, while having fewer extrapyramidal symptoms and side effects. They were also found to have better efficacy and results in regards to the negative symptoms of schizophrenia (1).

• 1896: Methylene blue is synthesized (1).
• 1933: France began to develop antihistamines (1,2)
• 1947: Promethazine was found to produce sedation and calmness in ani-mal models, and calmness in humans prior to surgery (1,2)
• 1950: Discovery of chlorpromazine, a derivative of promethazine. Chlor-promazine was also used for anesthesia (1,2).
• 1951: Chlorpromazine was found to have sedative properties (1).

- 1952: Chlorpromazine was used as a psychopharmacologic agent, and was found to make patients calmer, and used to treat things such as hallucinations and delusions (1,2).
- 1953: Further research was done confirming the efficacy of chlorpromazine (1). * 1955: Chlorpromazine was approved for antipsychotic use in the US, and then worldwide (1,2).
- 1960s: Explosion in the development of different antipsychotic drugs (1,2). Clozapine was found to have better response in the treatment of schizophrenia (1,2).
- 1972: Clozapine usage was introduced in Austria (1,2).
- 1974: Clozapine usage was introduced in Germany (1).
- 1990: Clozapine usage was approved in the US by the FDA (1).
- 1994: Risperidone approved in the US by the FDA (1).
- 1996: Olanzapine approved in the US by the FDA (1).
- 1997: Quetiapine approved in the US by the FDA (1).

The rich history of antipsychotic medications as well as its versatile use over time provides a neat segway into the advancements and modern uses of antipsychotics and how they have evolved.

# CHAPTER 2
## ADVANCEMENT AND MODERN USES OF ANTIPSYCHOTIC MEDICATIONS

### Peter Anto Johnson

The use of antipsychotic medications have advanced significantly over the years and are being prescribed much more frequently than it has been over a decade ago [1]. Currently, these medications are utilized to manage symptoms of psychosis, including delusions and hallucinations, mood stabilization in bipolar disorders, general management of schizophrenia, suicide prevention, anti-anxiety therapy, and in dementia/Alzheimer's disease management. In this chapter, the advances and contemporary uses of antipsychotics will be discussed.

### PSYCHOSIS MANAGEMENT

Antipsychotic medication can be used for symptom control in conditions that lead to psychosis (e.g., schizophrenia, bipolar disorder, Alzheimer's disease, and depression). Psychosis can be defined as a symptom that manifests and leads to a sense of detachment from reality. A few examples may include the patient experiencing feelings of grandeur, hallucinating sensations or sounds such as voices, footsteps or other noises, deluding themselves that there is someone pursuing them, or that they are under surveillance and being watched constantly.

### SCHIZOPHRENIA MANAGEMENT

For the management of schizophrenia, atypical or second-generation antipsychotics (with the exception of clozapine) are the first-line treatment options in most cases [2]. The immediate implementation of antipsychotic therapy is critical, most notably in the five years following the initial acute episode, as this is when there are the most major changes affecting the central nervous system. Over the course of the first week of treatment, the primary objective of antipsychotics is to mitigate aggressive behaviour and restore normal sleeping, eating, and other normal functions. Typically, monotherapy (i.e., a single medication) is used; however, in later stages of the disease, combination therapy may be considered.

The approach for the medical management of schizophrenia relies on the six stages of the Texas Medication Algorithm Project (TMAP) [2]. Stage 1 consists of monotherapy using an atypical antipsychotic, which would be followed by the Stage 2 combination therapy that adds either another atypical or typical antipsychotic if monotherapy is unresponsive. In the case that combination therapy is also unresponsive, TMAP Stage 3 involves the administration of clozapine, which is a potent atypical antipsychotic that could cause agranulocytosis or low white blood cell (WBC) counts. As a result, patients who are on TMAP Stage 3 therapy should have their WBC levels continuously monitored. Next in the sequence, TMAP Stage 4 consisting of clozapine combined with either an atypical or typical antipsychotic or in some cases, electroconvulsive therapy (ECT), should be considered if Stage 3 therapy is unresponsive. Following this, TMAP Stage 5 involving monotherapy with another antipsychotic drug can be considered if no response is elicited by Stage 4 therapies. Finally, TMAP Stage 6 management using a combination of antipsychotic therapies, ECT, and/or a mood stabilizer can be attempted.

### BIPOLAR DISORDERS MANAGEMENT

In bipolar disorder, antipsychotics are typically used for management of manic states, episodes, and symptoms [3]. They can also function as long-term mood stabilizers and are particularly useful when symptoms are severe or there are significant changes to behaviour. The starting dose of antipsychotics (normally atypical antipsychotics) in bipolar disorders are always low due to its well-recognized side effects, which include blurred vision, dry mouth, constipation, weight gain, and constellation of features observed in metabolic syndrome. As such, regular health check-ups at least every 3 months are a necessity and should be even more relevant and frequent if the patient is diabetic. Oftentimes, they can be combined with lithium and valproate.

Although there are numerous clinical guidelines and recommendations for the management of bipolar disorders, there are no algorithms like that developed for schizophrenia. As a result, the management of bipolar disorders with antipsychotics may be case-dependent and ultimately rely on the

9

availability, region, and resources of the healthcare setting. Nevertheless, many of the first-line therapies and approaches are similar involving mono-therapies initially, followed by combination therapy with other antipsychotics, other medications, and ECT.

## DEMENTIA/ALZHEIMER'S

Disease Management In patients with dementia or Alzheimer's disease, the use of antipsychotics has shown a modest efficacy in the management of psychosis, aggression, and agitation [4]. Unlike conditions such as schizophrenia and bipolar disorder, the administration of antipsychotic medication for patients with dementia or Alzheimer's disease is never the first-line therapy. In fact, their use in this population of patients is often restricted due to its adverse effects drug profile. These adverse effects include an increased risk of death, cerebrovascular adverse events (e.g., stroke, transient ischemic attacks, etc.), Parkinsonism (i.e., abnormal movements as seen in Parkinson's disease), sedation, alterations in gait, cognitive decline, and pneumonia. As a result, it is only in cases of severe symptoms where the patient has not responded to nonpharmacological treatments and other firstline management strategies that the use of antipsychotic agents should be considered. Nevertheless, over the past two decades, there has been a reported increase in the off-label use of antipsychotic medications despite warnings about its adverse effects.

## DEPRESSION MANAGEMENT

Perhaps the least recognized conditions which could involve the use of antipsychotic agents as therapy are depressive conditions; this is largely due to the role of antidepressants. Quite surprisingly for many, they can be used as a monotherapy or adjuvant therapy alongside antidepressants in the treatment of several depressive disorders - with or without psychosis and its related symptoms [5]. In fact, United States Food and Drug Administration (FDA) has approved atypical antipsychotics such as aripiprazole and quetiapine slow-release tablets as adjunctive treatment for depressive disorders and the combination of olanzapine (an atypical antipsychotic) and fluoxetine (a serotonin-selective reuptake inhibitor (SSRI) antidepressant medication) for management of treatment-resistant depression. In spite of this, it is vital to take precautions and monitor for any antipsychotic adverse effects including extrapyramidal symptoms, weight gain, and hyperglycemia.

## Mood Stabilization

In addition to its use in psychosis management, antipsychotic medications can also be utilized for mood stabilization. In many of the aforementioned conditions, these agents can serve both functions concurrently and thereby reduce the need for other mood stabilizing medications. For example, in bipolar disorder, antipsychotics can be effective in the initial stabilization of moods during manic episodes [6]. This is especially true because most mood stabilizer medications that are currently on the market are slow-acting and unable to achieve the desired effect within an acute period of time, which is often required for those patients experiencing significant disturbances in moods. Another example of its mood stabilizing effects is evidenced in the use of antipsychotics for the control of agitation, aggression, and hostile behaviour observed in patients with dementia and Alzheimer's disease or patients with intellectual disabilities who show this aggressive behaviour.

### Anti-anxiety Effects

Another promising use of antipsychotic therapy over the recent decades has been its use for the management of anxiety disorders [7]. While the FDA has already approved the use of typical antipsychotics for non-psychotic anxiety disorders, there has been a rise in the prescription and use of atypical anti-psychotics for managing anxiety in the recent decades - perhaps owing to its drug profile, which shows a relatively enhanced safety compared to typical antipsychotic agents. Although the body of literature evaluating the efficacy of atypical antipsychotics through rigorous randomized controlled trials is vastly different, there is moderately strong evidence that supports the utility of atypical antipsychotics in adjuvant therapy or monotherapy in treating non-psychotic anxiety. Despite this however, there are adverse side effects that must be considered before prescription and use for the majority of these patients with anxiety disorders. In fact, current data suggest that atypical antipsychotics should not be the first-line monotherapy or first- or second-line adjuvant treatment for the management of anxiety disorders. More studies are therefore warranted to support the off-label prescription and use of atypical antipsychotics for the treatment of anxiety disorder. At the same time, it is significant to note that patients who have severe anxiety disorder may indeed show an improvement if atypical antipsychotics are used as an adjunctive judiciously and with prudence. Thus, it is important that a physician undertakes a thorough cost-benefit analysis considering the risks and evaluating the patients on a case-by-case basis to determine the effectiveness of antipsychotic management for anxiety treatment.

## Suicide Prevention

Various properties and drug profiles of antipsychotic agents can have varying effects on suicidal thought and behaviour [8]. Generally, the atypical antipsychotics have been reported to have a greater potential for suicide prevention in patients who have schizophrenia, even though the relative profiles of each drug have yet to be calculated. For an antipsychotic to be effective in a patient who is at risk for suicide, it must be able to treat hostility, impulsivity, and depressive symptoms, while simultaneously not causing the extrapyramidal and metabolic syndrome-related side effects. Currently, there is the greatest body of evidence for the utilization of clozapine over any other atypical or typical antipsychotic for suicide prevention. Although this effect has not been demonstrated, the use of clozapine is recommended and particularly salient in patients who have schizophrenia and are suspected to be at a high risk for suicide to prevent ideation and action.

## Tic Management in Tourette Syndrome

An interesting application of atypical antipsychotic drugs has been its use for treating tics associated with Tourette Syndrome with comorbid psychiatric conditions [9]. Tourette's Syndrome is a neuropsychiatric disorder which begins in childhood and involves motor and verbal tics that vary throughout life. Although it may improve by the time the child has grown to late adolescence, occasionally some children and adults with Tourette's Syndrome can experience tic-related morbidity, which includes social and family relationship problems, academic challenges, and pain. If conservative interventions fail and psychiatric comorbidities challenge the management of Tourette's Syndrome, atypical antipsychotic therapy could be a promising second-line management strategy. Although there have been a few randomized controlled studies examining medications like risperidone, aripiprazole, and ziprasidone, unfortunately the body of evidence on the effectiveness and risks of atypical antipsychotic medications in the treatment of tics remain quite limited and there is only evidence to support a weak recommendation for its routine use in Tourette's Syndrome. Thus, more rigorous randomized clinical trials are warranted to better explore its role, clinical profile, and effects.

## Obsessive Compulsive Disorder Management

Although the first-line of treatment for Obsessive Compulsive Disorder (OCD) is the use of SSRIs, only 40-70% of patients respond to this therapy alone [10]. As a result, it is quite common to add antipsychotics to augment therapy for these patients. According to recent evidence, one of three patients that do not respond to SSRI treatment will show improvement with antipsychotic therapy augmentation. Of the antipsychotic agents, atypical antipsychotics including risperidone, and aripiprazole have the best evidence, whereas haloperidol is more uncertain clinical profile and second-line due to its adverse side effects. Ultimately, further studies with larger cohorts and more rigorous designs are necessitated for a comprehensive exploration and study of the use of antipsychotics in patients with OCD.

## POST TRAUMATIC STRESS DISORDER MANAGEMENT

Similar to OCD, evidence from randomized controlled trials have offered promise in the use of atypical antipsychotic medications for augmentation therapy in post-traumatic stress disorder (PTSD) patients [11]. Metabolic side effects including weight gain make antipsychotic therapies less appealing but clinical trials have shown potential with modest doses. In particular, several randomized controlled trials suggest the use of quetiapine monotherapy in military and non-military patients is effective in reducing PTSD symptoms. Notably however, these studies involved a small cohort and sample size. On the other hand, large-scale clinical trials have been performed examining augmentation therapy with atypical antipsychotics such as risperidone for PTSD showing small reductions in re-experiencing and hyperarousal symptoms. Many smaller trials demonstrated mixed results and focus extensively on combat-related PTSD. As a result, its generalizability to other types of PTSD is unclear and an area of research requiring further investigation.

## PERSONALITY DISORDER MANAGEMENT

Personality disorders, such as borderline personality disorder, is well-established for its increased rates of polypharmacy (i.e., use of multiple psychiatric medications at the same time) [12]. In fact, atypical antipsychotic medications are unofficially the mainstay for off-label prescription and medical management as there are no known medications indicated for its management. Unfortunately, strong evidence for the use of atypical antipsychotic medications is limited. While speculative, it has been proposed that atypical antipsychotics are useful for the management of symptoms such as depression, anxiety, anger, impulsivity, and paranoia/dissociative behavior characteristic of personality disorders.

Attention Deficit Hyperactivity Disorder (ADHD) is a condition that commonly affects children and youth, where atypical antipsychotics are a key management strategy in the recommendations [13]. Although much is not understood about the mechanism of action, numerous factors and comorbidities can also be reduced through antipsychotic treatment interventions. Numerous factors place ADHD patients at an increased risk, including other pharmacological medical treatments, self-harm/suicidal thoughts, defiant behaviour, substance use, depression, and anxiety disorder. As a result, the use of antipsychotic therapy may help reduce other mental health comorbidities but its overall role in ADHD management remains uncertain.

## INSOMNIA MANAGEMENT

The use of atypical antipsychotic medications for the management of insomnia is another novel field of study, which is filled with uncertainty [14]. Currently, atypical antipsychotics are not recommended as a first-line treatment in primary insomnia. According to observational studies, atypical antipsychotics such as quetiapine are increasingly being prescribed; however, the adverse effects and uncertainty are a cause of concern and ultimately suggest the need for a better classification of the sedative effects of antipsychotics. Although low quality evidence suggests a trend towards improvement in insomnia, a systematic review has suggested quetiapine does not significantly enhance sleep parameters and thus should not be recommended until further evidence is available.

## AUTISM SPECTRUM DISORDER AND PEDIATRIC INTELLECTUAL DISABILITY MANAGEMENT

For children with autism spectrum disorder, the use of atypical antipsychotic therapy has been approved by the FDA [15]. Many of the behavioural symptoms observed in autism can be managed through this therapy and its use as an adjuvant therapy alongside other drug classes such as antidepressants, anticonvulsants, and stimulants may be beneficial for diminishing aggression and irritability. Nevertheless, the efficacy of antipsychotic has yet to be clearly demonstrated and remains a weakly supported recommendation in the management of autism. A key limitation in the use of antipsychotics for autism are its side effects, which include weight gain, hyperprolactinemia, and tardive dyskinesia.

These side effects extend to other pediatric intellectual disabilities as well [16]. However, the vast majority of evidence in the literature about the use of antipsychotic medications remains poorly characterized. Meta-analyses have suggested that atypical antipsychotics could serve to reduce challenging behaviors in children with intellectual disabilities but at the same time, caution must be practiced in interpreting results from a limited dataset. In the end, the quality of evidence is low and there is an increased risk for many of the side effects - perhaps even more so in children who are more vulnerable than adults.

## OTHER USES

In addition to these, a number of other uses have also been implemented and suggested for antipsychotic medications in the literature including: prevention of schizophrenia, psychiatric conditions, treatment-resistant psychiatric conditions, and management of a number of developmental disorders. The latest technology in drug design and developments, modern research, and advancements have made it all the more possible to explore their uses and functions much more effectively than in the past.

# CHAPTER 3
## APPROVAL PROCESS AND LONGITUDINAL STUDIES EXPLORING THE USE OF THESE MEDICATIONS

## Sameen Ali

### INTRODUCTION

"My heart was shattered and every memory gathered was scattered across the sky like stars in dark matter." says Trevor Mills attempting to put into words what it is like to lose his brother – Spencer – to schizophrenia. Many people around the world resonate with Mills' story in various ways. Although there is no cure for this illness, it is widely treated and managed using antipsychotics. Antipsychotic medications are mainly used to treat patients with schizophrenia, psychosis which occurs in patients with bipolar disorder, depression and Alzheimer's disease (1). Psychosis affects the way the brain processes information; such complications result in a loss of touch in reality and patients may see, hear or believe things that are not real (2). Antipsychotic drugs aim to reduce such symptoms and also aims to reduce tics in tourette syndrome and anxiety in anxiety disorders (1). These are essential drugs that are vital to the lives of millions of people. However, it is essential to ensure that these drugs are safe and effective. How is this process accomplished?

To approve any type of medications, long term studies must be done. Health Canada is responsible for ensuring that the drug being approved is effective and safe for the public. All medications, including antipsychotic drugs must meet the requirements of the Food and Drug Act (3). The two branches within Health Canada that are responsible for ensuring these requirements are met are Therapeutic Products Directorate (TPD) or the Biologic and Genetic Therapies Directorate (BGTD) (3,5). The former is under the management of the Health Products and Food branch of Health Canada (3). The process requires intensive scientific testing followed by clinical trials. Even after approval, Canada continues to monitor the drugs effectiveness and side effects, they can remove approval at any time if complications arise or patients safety is at risk (3). However, to ensure that the use of antipsychotic drugs actually affects such diseases and symptoms, long term studies must be done. Let's look at such studies and see not only how these medications are established but also the exploration of longitudinal studies.

## APPROVAL PROCESS

Medications are only authorized once they have successfully completed the drug review process. This includes antipsychotic medication.This process is reviewed by scientists in the Health Products and Food Branch (HPFB) of Health Canada and also by outside experts to assess not only the efficacy of the medication but also safety and quality (4). Safety of citizens is kept number one priority and major concern throughout the entire process.The drug development process has been broken down into 5 stages: initial drug research, pre-clinical studies, clinical trials, the drug approval process and lastly, after approval (5).

## STAGE ONE

In the first stage – initial drug research – researchers begin by identifying chemicals and biological substances that will aid in the development of the desired drugs, in this case the desired drug would be antipsychotics. Many tests of multiple molecular compounds to find beneficial effects and use existing information on other medications that have effects are conducted (5). Once researchers have identified a promising compound, a plethora of tests to examine the activity, efficacy, and toxicity is conducted (5). The major goal of such tests is to gather information on its safety and effectiveness (5). For antipsychotics – depending on the type of antipsychotic medication these compounds would vary. For example, in seroquel – one of the most popular antipsychotic medications used for schizophrenia, bipolar disorder or major depressive disorder – one of the many biological compounds would consist of titanium dioxide (6). This compound would undergo the steps listed under stage one of the 5 stage cycle.

## STAGE TWO

After the completion of stage one, the preclinical studies stage begins. The next step is administering the drug to a selected species of animals or cells (5). The former refers to in vivo (when work is done within an entire living organism) and the latter as in vitro (work done outside the organism, this can include cells) (7). In order for this stage to be successfully executed, the drug must show no harm or serious side effects at the doses required to have an effect on the cell (5). If this step shows effectiveness further tests are conducted to further show its level of acceptability and safety in addition to its efficacy (5). If all these tests have positive outcomes then the next step in the approval process is to submit a Clinical Trial Application to the TPD or BGTP for authorization to allow for human participation in clinical trials (5). Drugs like antipsychotics that have been authorized to be marketed or sold in Canada must be studied in clinical trials. The results and information obtained from such trials have to be included in the relevant regulatory dossiers to be reviewed for the drug to eventually be authorized for sale in Canada by the HPFB (5). The results from the clinical trials conducted in humans are essential components of the review process. The main outcome from such trials is to gather clinical information about the drug's effectiveness, safety best determined by human use (5). It is also crucial to evaluate any drug reaction and compare the results to existing medications for similar disorders as the ones that are antipsychotic treatments. The medication is also often compared to a placebo (when no treatment is used).

STAGE THREE

When clinical trials have been completed the sponsor may choose to file a New Drug Submission with the HPFB in order to obtain authorization and sell the drug in Canada (5). However, when a sponsor conducts clinical trials in Canada, during the process a Clinical Trial Application (CTA) must be submitted to be reviewed and approved by the HPFB in order to proceed with trials (5). The results of these studies are essential as they are a part of the drug approval process. However, what exactly is a Clinical Trial Application? The Canadian CTA is simple and consists of documents such as administrative form, protocol, protocol summary, Informed Consent Form, Investigator's Brochure and quality dossier summary (5). These documents are reviewed by Health Canada and they notify the sponsor within 30 days. They may ask any questions that arose during the review process. If the HPFB provides authorization that's when the study is taken to the next step and done with human subjects. They are informed and have given their consent to the consequences and possible outcomes of the drug (5). The tests on these participants are conducted in controlled environments where the drug administration procedures and results are closely tracked and analyzed (5).

The clinical Trial consists of four phases – The Safety phase, The Effectiveness phase, The Confirmation Phase, and The Monitoring phase (5). Phase one usually tests the medication on a small group of healthy individuals for the first time. The purpose is to determine the correct dosage and determine what the drugs impact on the body is (5). It is also used to find reactions that may occur. In The Effective phase, a larger group of individuals with disorders that antipsychotic medication can treat is used. This is mainly to test the effectiveness of the drug (5). This stage can be long term. Phase three is the next step only if phase two had a positive outcome. The drug is given to an even larger group of patients and this is to confirm the effectiveness and monitor side effects. The last stage gathers more information on the best ways to use this drug, long term benefits and risks to the population when the medication is approved for administration (5).

## Stage Four

The Drug Approval Process is undergone when all clinical and preclinical trials indicate that the antipsychotic medication is clearly beneficial and that its risks are not outweighed by the benefits (5). The next step is to file a New Drug Submission (NDS) which will grant authorization to sell or prescribe it. The information that is part of the NDS application must be detailed enough that Health Canada can make an assessment on safety and effectiveness of the medication (5). Other documents like the common technical document which outlines the chemistry and manufacturing of the medication and the quality requirements (5). The HPFB reviews the NDS and all other documentation and information on the medication and evaluates the risks and benefits of the drug to the population (5). They also review packaging, labelling and manufacturing. This review process has a timeline of around 7 months to one year. Once the review is completed, if the benefits outweigh the risks and the side effects are manageable then the drug can be prescribed/sold (5).

## Stage Five

Getting approved isn't the last step of the process. Once the product is given to the patients that it was designed for, the HPFB requires that the use of the medication is done under the terms of its market authorization (5). Health Canada also requires updates such as new dosage forms, new strengths or any manufacturing changes (5). This step is ongoing but essential to ensuring patients safety. There are currently 10 different types of atypical antipsychotic medications that are being marketed in Canada (1). Let's specifically look at the clinical trials for antipsychotic medications and see what the emphasis of these tests are.

Most studies of new antipsychotic medications follow the traditional drug approval process. These studies focus on the reduction of symptoms such as hallucinations and delusions in patients with an illness or a poor response to a treatment (8). Secondary analysis which consists of a large number of participants have evaluated drug effects on various outcomes. Some other common symptoms include apathy and social withdrawal (8). Schizophrenia clinical trials involving antipsychotic medications draw a focus on efficacy in reducing psychotic symptoms and also relapse and rehospitalization (8). Such clinical trials have progressed in efficacy and effectiveness; however, these studies do not provide the information needed by doctors. Patient samples and conditions can affect the treatment response and the clinical outcome. Study samples for schizophrenia trials have generally included chronic patients with acute illness', patients who have poor responses to prior antipsychotics and patients with treatment resistant symptoms. These studies take 4-8 weeks in duration (8). During these studies there is a period without the antipsychotic drug of up to 7 days to avoid carryover effects of any prior antipsychotic medication the patient was using (8).

Neuropharmacology drugs – drugs that directly affect the nervous system – have a lower success rate in obtaining approval for each phase of the clinical drug development process compared with any other general medication (8). The nature of schizophrenia generates challenges for testing and the clinical process. This disease is purely symptomatic, each patient has a different case and it can get quite complex (8). This complexity arises from the fact that the amount of data collected in a trial is often large. In addition, participants are often difficult to recruit and drop out of these trials is often very common. This leads to incomplete datasets (8). Numerous investigation sites are required in order to have a large number of participants to identify clinically significant effects. All these components come together to create a challenge in achieving an understanding of effectiveness of current antipsychotic medication and propose challenges in the approval process (8).

## ETHICAL CONCERNS WITH ANTIPSYCHOTIC MEDICATION IN THE STAGE THREE – CLINICAL TRIALS

The use of placebo controls in schizophrenia trials is not preferred since the availability of effective antipsychotic drugs has been offered (8). There are several reasons why placebo control (using individuals who have schizophrenia but have not taken the new medication) is superior to active comparators (using individuals who have schizophrenia and have taken other medications similar to the one being studied). Placebo control allows for reliable evaluations (8). However, considering the risks of untreated psychosis in chronic schizophrenia, placebo-controlled trials are now only used for short periods and in safe settings such as patient units (8). For individuals who have experienced psychosis for the first time and achieve a decrease in the symptoms– a placebo controlled discontinuation study to help determine who might safely be able to discontinue medications might be justifiable for studying (8). An additional ethical concern that arises for schizophrenic trials is related to early treatment interventions (8). For example, in an individual who has prodromal symptoms – which refers to symptoms in the early stage – although early intervention can result in a positive outcome, the identification is difficulty and there might be considerable damage associated with a false-positive diagnoses for prodromal schizophrenia and may also result in exposure to antipsychotic medication when it was not required (8).

## LONGITUDINAL STUDIES EXPLORING THE USE OF ANTIPSYCHOTIC MEDICATION

### 20-YEAR STUDY TO DETERMINE IF ANTIPSYCHOTIC MEDICATIONS IMPACT SCHIZOPHRENIA

A long term assessment of antipsychotic medication was done on patients with schizophrenia. This follow up study was conducted on 139 patients suffering from illness (9). 70 of the patients had schizophrenia while 69 had mood disorders. These patients were followed up 6 times within a 20 year time period. The comparison between patients with schizophrenia prescribed the medication and patients who weren't was made (9). More specifically, the influence on work function was examined. While antipsychotic medications reduce psychosis for most patients with schizophrenia, four years later down the 20 year time frame, patients with schizophrenia who were not prescribed the medication have significantly better work functioning (9). The work performance of patients who were continuously prescribed antipsychotics at a low rate did not improve over time (9). Various other factors also interfered with the results. The follow ups occurred at 2 years, 2.5 years, 7.5 years, 10 years, 15 years, and 20 years. All patients with schizophrenia were diagnosed for more than 6 months (9). During the follow ups patients were assessed with research instruments for work functioning, and symptoms, rehospitalization, periods or recovery and antipsychotic drug treatment (9). Work function was assessed using a structured interview. Examples of the questions included "Are you employed at present?", "What jobs have you had?", "How long have you been employed."A scale from 1 to 5 was used on work functioning (9).

When examining patients with schizophrenia prescribed antipsychotic medication versus those who were not on medications displayed that there was no significant difference within the first follow up which was after 2 years (9). After this assessment, patients not on antipsychotics had a higher rate of employment. For the assessment after 4.5 years, 65% of the patients worked half-time or more (9). Unexpectedly, the individuals who were not on the medication worked more. 9 of 36 patients with schizophrenia who were prescribed medications were working compared to 16 of 22 schizophrenia patients who were not prescribed any (9). In general, patients with schizophrenia who were continuously prescribed antipsychotics were significantly more likely to have negative symptoms than those not prescribed any at the 4.5 year followup mark (9). Negative symptoms are when patients appear to withdraw from the world around them and appear emotionless; in contrast, positive symptoms are changes in behavior or thoughts such as hallucinations or delusions (10). After the first follow up, patients with schizophrenia with negative symptoms were less likely to be working in the next follow-ups (9). Negative symptoms are a hindrance to work; the data indicated that at the 2 year follow ups only 2 schizophrenia patients were working (9).

Psychosis is an important measure of illness when it comes to schizophrenia. The comparison of schizophrenia patients with psychosis allows comparison of work functioning (9). Psychosis was a strong influence on work adjustment after 2-year follow ups. At the last follow up, which happened after 4.5 to 20 years, patients with schizophrenia and psychosis symptoms showed worse work function than patients who did not have the symptoms (9). After 2 years assessment more than 60% of the patients who did not have psychosis symptoms were working half-time or more (9).

Recent works from such longitudinal studies have displayed that there is still not a strong positive effect of treatment with antipsychotic medication beyond the first 3 initial years of usage of the medication. Many have questioned its long-term efficacy (9). Many negative outcomes from long term studies have been displayed (9). Longitudinal studies have not shown positive effects for patients with schizophrenia who are prescribed antipsychotic medication for long periods of time. Other studies similar to this have raised questions about long term necessity of antipsychotic medications (9). This is an area that is being studied to further understand the details.

The use of antipsychotic medication is high among long-term care (LTC) residents yet little is known about the correlation of such drugs and settings such as LTC (11). A study done investigated the frequency and correlation of new medication used on newly admitted LTC residents (11). This data was used from the interRAI Nursing Home (11). The data about demographics, clinical, medical and social use was collected in Ontario, Canada and obtained from provincial repositories at the University of Waterloo (11). In the data, follow up assessments were made after a maximum of 180 days. Residents were classified into groups that use antipsychotics, new users who have recently been prescribed the medication after the follow-up, continuous users and discontinuous users who started using the medication but stopped during follow ups. The presence of health conditions such as dementia, diabetes, congestive heart failure and hypertension was also considered.

The results displayed that new users were significantly more cognitively impaired than non users. Although behaviour problems were common, they were more prominent in new users (11). Compared to non-users, new users of antipsychotics reported more communication problems and higher rates of dementia, depressive symptoms, delusions and restlessness (11). In addition, social interaction was lower for new users than non users. New users also suffered more behavioural issues and conflicts with staff and family. New users were reported to be more isolated, and health status instability was higher in new users. Because of these shocking results, both the Food and Drug Administration (FDA) and European Medicine Agency (EMA) have issued official warnings to limit the use of these medications (11). A separate study done also displayed the increase of antipsychotic medication use in transitioning from community to institutional settings (11). These findings give insight into patterns of prescribing medications in institutional settings. Such longitudinal studies display essential implications for public health policy (11).

## CONCLUSION

Although the approval process for antipsychotic is more challenging than any other drug and may propose ethical dilemmas. It is important to overcome them in order to prevent more heart wrenching stories like Trevor Mills' to come to life. The process is long yet essential, each phase and stage plays an important role in the safety and efficacy of the drug. In addition to the long process, it is essential to have longitudinal studies. Such studies help with understanding if the drug is effective and how the patient's life is impacted. Since antipsychotics are famously used for schizophrenia, long term studies like the one conducted over a 20 year time frame are important to seeing exactly which factors in specific are impacted. Longitudinal studies also display that in addition to clinical factors, behaviour and social characteristics is also associated with antipsychotic medication use upon admission into facilities such at LTC homes. Such knowledge can bring insight into identifying targets for intervention to increase quality of care, especially in the elderly. Reducing inappropriate usage if antipsychotic medication is the goal and to improve the lives of many.

# CHAPTER 4
# WHAT ARE THE INDICATIONS OF USE FOR EACH TYPICAL AND ATYPICAL ANTIPSYCHOTIC MEDICATION

## Nasia Sheikh

Antipsychotic medications, also referred to as neuroleptics or major tranquilizers, are primarily used to manage psychosis (1,2). Psychosis refers to conditions that affect the mind in such a way that there is some loss of contact with reality (1). This includes delusions as well as hallucinations. People who experience psychosis can become a danger to themselves and others (2). Common mental disorders that fall under this term are schizophrenia, bipolar disorder, attention deficit hyperactivity disorder, post-traumatic stress disorder, obsessive compulsive disorder, and psychotic depression (1). Antipsychotic medications are also often prescribed to treat and reduce symptoms associated with senile psychoses, organic psychoses, and drug-induced psychoses and can have both short-term sedative and long-term effects (2). It is important to note that antipsychotic medications do not cure any of the above listed conditions, they are used to help relieve symptoms and improve quality of life (1).

There are many types of antipsychotic drugs that are available in oral dosage forms such as, tablets, dry powder, and capsules, as well as in parenteral forms such as, intramuscular and intravenous injections (2). Antipsychotic drugs can be classified into two groups: typical and atypical. This distinction is based off the drugs ability to cause extrapyramidal side effects such as dystonia (muscle spasm or contraction), akathisia (motor restlessness), or dyskinesia (irregular muscle movement), which is more common in typical antipsychotic drugs (3). These two classes also differ in their mechanism of action and metabolic side effects (3).

Typical antipsychotic drugs, which are also considered "first generation" antipsychotic drugs were first developed in the 1950s (2). This class of antipsychotic drugs is used in the treatment of severe psychosis when newer medications are ineffective, but they are associated with many side effects, some being quite severe (2). Due to the high risk of side effects, another class of antipsychotic drugs was developed, identified as atypical, or "second generation", antipsychotic drugs (2). Atypical antipsychotic drugs were first approved for use in the 1990's and typically are less likely to produce extrapyramidal effects, even at clinically effective doses (2).

## TYPICAL ANTIPSYCHOTIC DRUGS

Typical antipsychotic drugs are generally weaker in treating cognitive impairment compared to atypical (3). There are four common typical antipsychotic drugs: Chlorpromazine, Haloperidol, Perphenazine, and Fluphenazine (1). Each have their own distinct mechanism of action, indication of use, and side effects. Haloperidol Haloperidol is the most common typical antipsychotic drug used in treating patients with both acute and chronic schizophrenia (4). Schizophrenia is a complex and debilitating neuropsychiatric disorder (5). There are two common manifestations of schizophrenia: (1) 'positive' symptoms such as fixed, false beliefs (delusions) and perceptions without cause (hallucinations); and (2) 'negative' symptoms such as apathy and lack of drive, disorganization of behaviour and thought, and catatonic symptoms (6). The degree of suffering and disability is extreme, with over 80% of patients diagnosed with schizophrenia not being able to work and up to 10% dying by suicide (6). Haloperidol is also used to control tics and vocal utterances of Tourette's disorder in children and adults and is effective in treating patients with severe behavioural problems (4). This includes patients, especially children, with combative, explosive hyper-excitability, as well as hyperactive children who show excessive motor activity associated with impulsivity, difficulty in sustaining attention, aggression, and poor frustration tolerance (4). Haloperidol is also used to treat delirium (7). Haloperidol is a lipophilic compound, indicating increased ability to combine or dissolve in lipids or fats, therefore is easily metabolized in humans (4). Due to this, haloperidol has high inter-individual variability. Haloperidol has a narrow therapeutic window, therefore, requiring individualised optimisation for each patient (4).

Haloperidol is administered intravenously, intramuscularly, or orally to patients with schizophrenia (4). Intramuscular injection is the preferred route when treating acute schizophrenia as it leads to the immediate control of patients with psychosis-related violent behaviour (4). When ingesting haloperidol to maintain therapy, the oral route is preferred (4).

Although Haloperidol is highly effective in treating schizophrenia, it is still a typical, first generation antipsychotic drug, thus it is associated with severe extrapyramidal side effects (8). These side effects include primarily dystonia, but also constipation, dry mouth, blurred vision, urine hesitancy, sexual dysfunction, and some evidence to suggest a relationship with sudden death (8).

## CHLORPROMAZINE

Chlorpromazine (CPZ) was introduced in the early 1950s and catalyzed the development of psychopharmacology as well as improved understanding of chemical signaling in neurotransmission (9). It is used primarily to treat schizophrenia. Prior to CPZ, diagnosis of schizophrenia entailed confinement to an asylum for life and treatment included electroconvulsive therapy (9). CPZ also aided in reducing the stigma surrounding mental illness, which subsequently led to the deinstitutionalization of patients with schizophrenia (9).

Chlorpromazine was originally developed in 1952 to reduce allergic reactions before being used (in combination with other drugs) to induce a state of 'artificial hibernation' for surgery (10). The drug's ability to reduce psychic stress led researchers to believe that it could also be effective in treating psychiatric disorders (10). Thus leading to the discovery that CPZ was effective in treating schizophrenia. As this was the first drug to effectively treat schizophrenia, it was regarded as a revolution in psychiatry, second to the discovery of psychoanalysis (10).

CPZ was the first of many drugs that were later classified as neuroleptic – to grasp the nerve (10). It produces antipsychotic effects by acting on particular areas within specific cells in the brain (10). It is believed that CPZ affects the receptivity of these cells to dopamine, but it's effects are not specific to one site in the body, which leads to adverse effects in other areas of the body (10). These include dry mouth, blurred vision, tremors, facial rigidity, repetitive movements, and has even been associated with a potentially fatal disturbance of blood pressure, temperature, and muscle control (10). CPZ is one of the most common and inexpensive 'typical' antipsychotic drug treatments for patients with schizophrenia (10). However, there are well-documented, severe side effects associated with the use of CPZ. Despite this, it is still listed as one of the essential drugs by the World Health Organization (10).

Perphenazine is another type of typical antipsychotic drug. It was first formulated in the 1950s and distributed as an oral medication in late 1957, and as an injectable intravenous or intramuscular treatment in the 1970s (11). Perphenazine is primarily used now to treat schizophrenia but can also be used to treat other psychiatric disorders such as mania, agitated behaviour, and severe anxiety (11). This drug has also been shown to be effective in managing post-operative or chemotherapy-induced nausea and vomiting (11).

Schizophrenia is a chronic disorder that is believed to be caused by hyper-dopaminergic states in the limbic system (12). Therefore, antipsychotic drugs are targeted at blocking dopamine receptors. Perphenazine is a phenothiazine antipsychotic that effectively treats the positive symptoms of schizophrenia (hallucinations and delusions) (12). It has neuroleptic properties, thus it has extrapyramidal adverse effects (11). The concentration of perphenazine is greatly reduced before it reaches the systemic circulation, also referred to as the 'first-pass effect', making its bioavailability only about 40 percent (11). Only 2 percent of the absorbed perphenazine is excreted by urine in the non-metabolized form (11).

Perphenazine is less potent than haloperidol but approximately five times more potent than chlorpromazine, thus it is considered a medium potency antipsychotic drug (12). It does, however, share the side effects of haloperidol, including the extrapyramidal side effects (12).

### ATYPICAL ANTIPSYCHOTIC DRUGS

Atypical antipsychotic drugs are antipsychotic drugs that result in minimal extrapyramidal side effects at a clinically effective dose (3). This definition originated after observing that chlorpromazine, a typical antipsychotic drug, as well as other selective dopamine D2 receptor antagonist-based antipsychotic drugs resulted in extrapyramidal side effects, such as tardive dyskinesia, which may become fatal, and neuroleptic malignant syndrome (3). These side effects are likely a result of a blockade of dopamine receptors in the limbic region of the brain (3).

There are two classes of atypical antipsychotic drugs that are currently widely used and several in development (3). The larger of the two classes consist of drugs that are more potent 5-HT2A receptor antagonists effective-

28

ly blocking serotonin reuptake, than antagonists of dopamine D2 receptors (3). The atypical antipsychotic drugs in clinical use from this class includes clozapine, asenapine, blonanserine, iloperidone, lurasidone, melperone, paliperidone, quetiapine, risperidone, ziprasidone, and zotepine (3). The second class of atypical antipsychotic drugs are believed to be D2/D3 receptor antagonists, but many of the drugs in this class also have serotonergic effects (3). These include amisulpride, a potent 5-HT7 antagonist, and cariprazine, a potent 5-HT2B antagonist and 5-HT1A partial antagonist (3). Other D2/D3 receptor antagonist atypical drugs also have a variety of serotonergic actions, thus the distinction between these two classes of atypical drugs is not absolute (3).

## CLOZAPINE

Clozapine is considered the "gold standard" of atypical antipsychotic drugs due to its high efficacy in treating positive symptoms in treatment-resistant schizophrenia (3). The success of clozapine established an expectation that all atypical antipsychotic drugs would have similar effects, which was ultimately discovered to not be the case (3).

Clozapine was the first antipsychotic drug shown to be effective in treating psychotic symptoms in treatment-resistant schizophrenia patients and is still the only approved drug for treatment-resistant schizophrenia (3). The response rate in patients have been shown to be effective up to 6 weeks into treatment by clozapine, with some patients seeing results 6 months into treatment (3). Some advantages of clozapine over other atypical and typical antipsychotic drugs are that it decreases aggressiveness and violence in psychiatric patients, controls psychosis in Parkinson's disease, and reduces the risk of developing tardive dyskinesia, while also treating it (3).

Clozapine is also associated with reducing the risk for suicide in patients with schizophrenia (3). This drug is also useful for patients with schizophrenia who are not able to tolerate other antipsychotic drugs due to extrapyramidal side effects (3). However, clozapine has a myriad of other side effects including agranulocytosis, eosinophilia, and fever at treatment onset, as well as metabolic side effects including hyperlipidosis, type 2 diabetes, and weight gain (3). This drug may also result in major motor and myoclonic seizures, myocarditis, hypersalivation, urinary incontinence, and constipation (3). These side effects have resulted in clozapine being underutilized in the United States despite these side effects rarely requiring discontinuation of treatment, with the exception of agranulocytosis and myocarditis (3).

Olanzapine is an atypical antipsychotic that is used in the treatment of schizophrenia and has been shown to some degree to effectively improve negative and cognitive symptoms (13). Schizophrenia is a severe mental disorder with clinical presentation including positive, negative, and cognitive symptoms, which can result in significant disability (13). Specifically, cognitive impairments are a core feature of schizophrenia and a predictor of reduced function, whereas deficits in emotion processing underlie negative symptoms and interfere with inter and intrapersonal functions (13). Olanzapine has a higher affinity for serotonin than dopamine receptors at histaminergic, adrenergic, and muscarinic binding sites (13). It is one of the most commonly prescribed atypical antipsychotic drugs due to its efficacy in combatting positive and negative symptoms of schizophrenia as well as its positive effects on cognitive deficits (13). The exact mechanism by which olanzapine produces its antipsychotic effects has not yet been elucidated, but the current proposed mechanism is that it is mediated through dopamine (D2) and serotonin (5-HT2) antagonism (14). Despite not knowing the exact mechanism of action, olanzapine has UD Food and Drug Administration (FDA) approval for acute and maintenance treatment of schizophrenia and bipolar disorder (14). Olanzapine may also be used in treatment of agitation related to delirium, dementia, or substance intoxication as well as other psychotic disorders including major depressive disorder with psychosis, and chemotherapy-induced nausea and vomiting (14).

Olanzapine can be administered orally, through tablets and through intramuscular injection (14). There are two forms of intramuscular olanzapine: an immediate release and a long-acting form. The long-acting intramuscular medication is generally used for maintained treatment of schizophrenia and administered every 2 to 4 weeks, while the immediate release intramuscular medication is used for the management of acute agitation (14).

Additionally, although clozapine is the only approved drug for treatment-resistant schizophrenia, there is evidence that suggests that high doses of olanzapine may also be effective in treating treatment-resistant schizophrenia (3). This could be due to the fact that olanzapine is the closest atypical antipsychotic drug that is pharmacologically similar to clozapine (3). AripiprazoleAripiprazole was the first atypical antipsychotic drug developed that possessed dopamine D2 autoreceptor agonist properties, which has provided a new avenue for schizophrenia drug discovery (15). Earlier antipsychotic medications were dopamine D2 antagonists, which resulted in dopamine receptor blockades. Extensive dopamine receptor blockade, however, typically results in extrapyramidal side effects, which was a major disadvantage of the first generation (typical) antipsychotic drugs (15). Second generation antipsychotics, such as clozapine, had significantly lower risk for extrapyramidal side effects, but had an abundance of other side effects such as metabolic dysfunction and weight gain (15). Aripiprazole however, has been shown to successfully reduce positive, negative, and cognitive symptoms of schizophrenia, while also minimizing risk of weight gain and extrapyramidal side effects (15). A disadvantage of aripiprazole, however, is that it has been linked to compulsive behaviours in a small group of schizophrenia patients (15).

Aripiprazole functions by binding dopamine receptors with a greater affinity compared to other antipsychotics (16). Compared to aripiprazole, haloperidol binds with less affinity to the dopamine receptor (16). Aripiprazole however, binds to opioid, norepinephrine, serotonin, benzodiazepine, and muscarinic receptors with low affinity (16). This drug acts as a partial agonist and stabilizer at the dopamine D2 receptor and binds in its G-protein-coupled state, thereby blocking the receptor in the presence of excessive dopamine (16). Aripiprazole fulfills the role of a stabilizer by stimulating the receptor when there is no excess dopamine, which is different from haloperidol which acts purely as a dopamine antagonist (16). This leads to lower risk of extrapyramidal side effects, sedation, and elevation in serum prolactin levels by aripiprazole compared to other antipsychotics (16).

Aripiprazole can be administered orally, intramuscularly, and intravenously. With oral ingestion, peak plasma concentrations occur within 3 to 5 hours with 87% bioavailability (16). With intramuscular administration, there is greater absorption compared to oral ingestion with plasma concentrations reaching 78% of maximum concentration within 30 minutes of injection and a 98% bioavailability (16). Conclusion   In conclusion, there are two major types of antipsychotic medications, typical and atypical. Typical antipsychotics are considered first-generation, as they were discovered before atypical antipsychotics. They are typically associated with high risk of extrapyramidal side effects, while atypical antipsychotics are not. Both groups have a few different types of medications, each with their own individual costs and benefits. Determining which medication is best for patients may vary from patient to patient, and although one may be successful in treating one patient, it may not be for another. Patients should consult with a physician before deciding which antipsychotic drug is the best fit for them.

# CHAPTER 5
## ADVERSE EFFECTS OF ANTIPSYCHOTICS AND THE ADDICTIVENESS AND DEPENDENCY

### By Justine Nicole Banszky

Psychosis is a disorder that can appear in a number of different psychiatric disorders. The most commonly known ones are schizophrenia, schizophrenic bipolar personality disorder, bipolar disorder, and it can even appear in people without the previous listed disorders (1). Typically, an episode of psychosis happens when a person loses touch with reality and that can be identified as having hallucinations, periods of delusion, incoherent speech, and can lead a person to behave in a way that is not appropriate for the situation they are in (2). A person suffering from an episode of psychosis will understandably be confused by their surroundings and not be able to understand what is going on around them. They are removed from reality and the effects of that can lead to a state of depression, on-going anxiety, problems with sleep and rest, social withdrawal, and over all struggle with functioning in the day-to-day mundanity of life (2). Thankfully, modern technology has led to the development of antipsychotic medication that helps to manage and control symptoms of psychosis. However, like with all medications, antipsychotics can have adverse side effects and can affect users in different ways, and can even lead to cases of dependency (1).

Antipsychotic drugs have gone through two generations of development. The first generations of antipsychotic drugs came into development in the 1950's and 60's and includes: Benperidol (Anquil), Chlorpromazine (Largactil), Flupentixol (Depixol), Fluphenazine (Modecate), Haloperidol (Haldol), Levomepromazine (Nozinan), Pericyazine, Perphenazine (Fentazin), Pimozide (Orap), Promazine, Sulpiride (Dolmatil, Sulpor), Zuclopenthixol (Clopixol) (1).

# FIRST-GENERATION

## BENPERIDOL

Benperidol is a first-generation antipsychotic medication developed to treat dementia and psychosis in adults, as well as for controlling anti-social sexual behaviour and social deviants (3). A dose is taken through oral ingestion and is considered highly toxic when inhaled (3). extrapyramidal symptoms such as tremor, rigidity, hypersalivation, bradykinesia, akathisia, acute dystonia, oculogyric crisis and laryngeal dystonia might occur in the patient (3). Other adverse side effects include rare cases of sudden and unexplained death in those with a history of cardiac diseases, uncorrected electrolyte disturbances, and pointes (3). Benperidol is not considered an addictive drug, however the withdrawal symptoms (nausea, vomiting, and insomnia) could make it difficult for a patient to stop taking the medication (3).

## CHLORPROMAZINE

Chlorpromazine is another first-generation antipsychotic medication that was developed for the treatment of nausea, vomiting, and schizophrenia (4). In some cases, Chlorpromazine is also used to settle a person's nerves prior to surgery, hiccups, behaviour problems in children under twelve years of age, and to help with manic-depressive illness (4).

An adverse reaction to watch out for is agranulocytosis, which is a very low white blood cell count, and other blood dyscrasias including haemolytic anaemia and thrombocytopenia (5). Chlorpromazine has also been known to impair the patient's ability to regulate their body temperature and affect the body's ability to process glucose (5). Like many antipsychotic medications, Chlorpromazine is not considered to have addictive qualities, however, withdrawal symptoms such as nausea, vomiting, and insomnia have been reported and cane cause a difficult transition away from the medication, it is advised that a person gradually withdraws from the medication (5).

## FLUPENTIXOL

Flupentixol, also known as Depixol, is used in the treatment of chronic schizophrenic episodes in patients who do not usually experience agitation, excitement, or hyperactivity as a symptom, as well as other forms of psychosis (6). Secondly, this medication can be used in the treatment of depression and depression induced anxiety (6). There are two ways that a person can receive their dose which have different effects on the amount of time the drug stays active in the body before a new dose is needed: oral or injection (7). An injection will stay in the body for up to three weeks before another dose is needed whereas the tablet starts to become fully metabolized after 35 hours (6).

Adverse reactions to the medication include a higher risk of developing neuroleptic malignant syndrome (7) a condition that can cause fever and an altered start of reality, along with muscle spasms (8). Flupentixol, like most antipsychotic medications, is not considered to have addictive qualities, however, the body can become dependent on the medication and cause withdrawal symptoms (7). Withdrawal symptoms such as nausea, vomiting, sweating and insomnia have been reported and it is best to slowly withdraw from the medication (7).

## HALOPERIDOL

Haloperidol, a first-generation antipsychotic medication is used in the treatment of schizophrenia, agitation, irritability, delirium, and other modes of psychosis (9). It is considered to be very successful in treating the "positive" symptoms of psychosis such as outburst of anger, hearing voices, hallucinations, and disorganized speech (9). Haloperidol is trusted world-wide and is one of the more popular prescribed medications (9). Haloperidol offers a high potency and combats psychosis by targeting the dopamine receptors in the brain (9). Like most antipsychotic medications, it can also be used to treat other conditions, in this particular case, Haloperidol can be used to treat side effects of Tourette's syndrome and Huntington's disease (10).
Adverse side effects include rare but sudden death, depression, poor metabolism as well as having negative effects on Cardiovascular health (10). It is considered a rare adverse side effect but issues with arrhythmias can occur and is more common in patients with pre-existing cardiovascular health issues (10). Another adverse side effect is seizures and convulsions and therefore should be avoided by patients with a history of epilepsy (10). Haloperidol is not considered to be addictive, however when taken regularly the body can become dependent on the drug and cause withdrawal symptoms such as vomiting, nausea, and insomnia (10).

## LEVOMEPROMAZINE

Levomepromazine, more commonly known as Nozinan, is a first-generation antipsychotic medication designed for the treatment of schizophrenia and for manic phases of bipolar disorder (11). Due to its nature and histamine-antagonist properties, Levomepromazine can also work as a sedative and has been used to treat terminally ill patients (12). Adverse side effects include, fatigue, stroke, increased chance of sudden death in elderly patients, hyperglycaemia, convulsions, and venous thromboembolism (VTE) (12).

Levomepromazine is not considered to be addictive, however when taken regularly the body can become dependent on the drug and cause withdrawal symptoms such as vomiting, nausea, and insomnia (12).

### PERICYAZINE

Pericyazine is unique in that it is prescribed as a companion drug to other prescriptions to treat impulsive and aggressive behaviours in psychosis conditions, such as bipolar disorder and schizophrenia, by creating a central adrenergic blockade (13). When taking Pericyazine, aggression and impulsivity can be treated without contributing to an abnormal mental integration (13). However, that does not mean that Pericyazine does not have adverse side effects. Some adverse side effects are upset stomach, nausea and gastrointestinal issues with people that have lactose intolerance (14). In other patents, adverse effects include low blood count, seizures, unexplained fevers, sweating and artery instability, and stroke (14). All adverse side effects can be worsened by taking Pericyazine with other neuroleptics such as Agomelatine, aclidinium, and acetophenazine, which all can contribute to increase in seizures and in some cases hypertension (13).

Addiction in not typically associated with Pericyazine and it is not considered to have addictive properties, however when taken regularly the body can and will become dependent on the drug and cause withdrawal symptoms such as vomiting, nausea, insomnia, and in cases, with people pro to seizures are at risk of having seizures and convulsions (14).

### PERPHENAZINE

Perphenazine is another first-generation antipsychotic drug used in the treatment of schizophrenia, anxiety, varying degrees of depression, and agitation (15). Interestingly, Perphenazine was also developed to treat excessive vomiting and nausea in adults (15). Perphenazine, like most medication developed for the treatment of psychosis, Perphenazine targets the dopamine receptors, but it is different from some others because it works with the nervous system:

Perphenazine is a piperazinyl phenothiazine, acts on the central nervous system, and has a greater behavioral potency than other phenothiazine derivatives whose side chains do not contain a piperazine moiety. It is a member of a class of drugs called phenothiazines, which are dopamine D1/D2 receptor antagonists. Perphenazine is 10 to 15 times as potent as chlorpromazine; that means perphenazine is a highly potent antipsychotic. In equivalent doses it has approximately the same frequency and severity of early and late extrapyramidal side-effects compared to Haloperidol. (15)

Adverse side effects to Perphenazine can include convulsive seizures in children and can cause liver failure in adults that have liver disease (15). Perphenazine can be dangerous when taken with other medications, such as Acebutolol, which will increase the serum level of Perphenazine in the body causing toxicity which can lead to seizures and a comatose state (15). Another adverse side effect is that Perphenazine can increase the effects of alcohol and therefore should not be mixed with alcoholic beverages as it can lead the user to higher levels of intoxication (15).

PIMOZIDE

Pimozide was developed during the first-generation of antipsychotic medication to treat symptoms of psychosis in adults and has the added benefit of making debilitating motor and phonic tics in patients with Tourette's Disorder manageable (16). The reason Pimozide is effective in treating both psychosis and tics associated with Tourette's' Disorder is because it inhibits the dopamine D2 receptors in the central nervous system (16). Pimozide is an effective antipsychotic agent that causes less, however, like most medications Pimozide can affects the body in adverse ways such as prolonging the QT interval, depression, and increase in mortality in the elderly with dementia, ventricular arrhythmias, and toxicity in the liver (17).

Withdrawal symptoms will always vary from person to person; however, it is documented that for patients with schizophrenia the treatment might be delayed and if the drug is withdrawn there could be a delay in the symptoms representing themselves to the patient (17). An abrupt halt to taking Pimozide can result in adverse withdrawal symptoms such as nausea, vomiting, insomnia, psychotic symptoms may return or reoccur, and involuntary movement disorders might also present themselves in the patient (17).

Promazine is primarily used in the short-term treatment of schizophrenia and disturbed behaviour as an antiemetic and can also be used to treat agitation and violent behaviour in the elderly (18). Promazine manages to control symptoms of psychosis and restlessness by blocking the dopamine receptors in the brain and prevents them from overstimulating the brain and therefore prevents the ongoing effects of psychotic illness (18). However, Promazine is not considered to be suitable for long term treatment as it is a weaker form of antipsychotic medication (18).

Adverse side effects are rather limited, however, those with pre-existing liver diseases of respiratory diseases are at risk of furthering their conditions (19). Prolonged use of Promazine in the elderly may cause dyskinesias, and in children there is a risk of akathisia as well as dyskinesias (19). Other adverse effects include prolactin secretion, hypothyroidism, and pheochromocytoma (19). Like most antipsychotics, Promazine is not documented as possessing addictive qualities, however, withdrawal symptoms such as nausea, vomiting, sweating, and insomnia can make it difficult for a patient to come off the medication (19).

## SULPIRIDE

Sulpiride first appeared on the market in 1967 and was developed for the treatment of chronic and acute schizophrenia (20). Studies showed that Sulpiride was effective in treating the negative symptoms opposed to the positive symptoms in schizophrenic patients (20). The medication is not approved for use in North America and is only availed in select European countries (20). Adverse side effects include aggression, agitation, inability to control feelings of excitement, sedation, confusion, weight gain, stroke, akathisia, breast cancer, and in some cases fatality (21). Addictive qualities and withdrawal symptoms are not known (21).

## ZUCLOPENTHIXOL

Approved for use in Canada in 2011, Zuclopenthixol is a thioxanthene-based neuroleptic antipsychotic drug used in the treatment of schizophrenia (22). Zuclopenthixol primary mode of action is by antagonising the D1 and D2 dopamine receptors in the brain (22). Adverse side effects in children are unknown as studies in children have not been approved, however, adverse side effects in adults include muscle spasms and rigidity, liver disease, heart disease, and arrythmias (23). Like most antipsychotic medications, Zuclo-penthixol has been designed to not have any addictive qualities, however, withdrawal symptoms such as nausea, vomiting, insomnia, muscle spasms, and sweating can make it difficult for a person to remove the medication from their life (23).

Second-generation antipsychotic drugs began appearing on the market in the early 1990s (2). They are considered to be more effective and have fewer side effects when compared to the first generation of antipsychotic medi-cations (2). Like the first-generation of medications, the second-generation work by helping the brain to carry messages from one part of the brain to the other and help to reduce the amount of dopamine produced in the brain or to inhibit the dopamine receptors in the brain (2). The list of second-generation medications include: Amisulpride (Solian) Aripiprazole (Abilify, Abilify Maintena Clozapine (Clozaril, Denzapine, Zaponex) Risperidone (Risperdal & Risperdal Consta) Olanzapine (Zyprexa) Quetiapine (Seroquel) (2).

### Second-generation

#### Amisulpride

Amisulpride is a second-generation antipsychotic medication that can be used in the treatment of both positive and negative symptoms of schizophre-nia (24). Amisulpride works by inhibiting the dopamine production in the D2 and D3 dopamine receptors in the brain as well as working preferentially in the limbic system (25). Amisulpride has not been properly tested for the use of children under the age of 18 and is also not recommended for patients over the age of 65 (24). Not all medications have the same side effects, nor do side effects appear in all patients. However, adverse side effects to watch out for include high levels of liver toxicity, muscle rigidity and autonomic instability, stroke, and akathisia (24). However, with most second-generation medications the chances of experiencing adverse side effects is more rare (2). Antipsychotic medications, such as Amisulpride, have been designed to not have any addictive qualities, however, withdrawal symptoms such as nausea, vomiting, insomnia, muscle spasms, and sweating can make it diffi-cult for a person to remove the medication from their life (23). The best way to avoid withdrawal symptoms is to gradually withdraw from the medication and the body slowly to lose its dependency on the medication (24).

# ARIPIPRAZOLE

Aripiprazole is capable of treating a variety of mood and psychotic disorders including Tourett's syndrome, bipolar disorder, schizophrenia, and irritability that can present itself in people with autism (26).

Mechanism for action:

> The antipsychotic action of aripiprazole is likely due to the agonism of D2 and 5-HT1A receptors though the exact mechanism has not been defined. Some adverse effects may be due to action on other receptors. For example, orthostatic hypotension may be explained by antagonism of the adrenergic alpha1 receptors (26)

Unfortunately, Aripiprazole comes with some adverse side effects such as suicidal tendencies, cardiovascular health issues, seizures, weight gain, hypersensitivity, dysphagia, moto abilities leading to increase chance of falling and collapsing, and it can cause an increase in mortality in the elderly (27). Further, the medication contains a mixture of sucrose and fructose sugars and can cause harm to the patients' teeth if not handled correctly (27). When medication is stopped abruptly it can cause an episode of 'rebound psychosis' where the patients' symptoms can occur in a high quantity (2). Addictiveness is not associated with Aripiprazole but with most antipsychotic medications the body does become dependent, and withdrawal needs to be done gradually (27).

# CLOZAPINE

Clozapine is unique in the way that it is prescribed to patients with psychosis (2). First off, it is considered a 'last-resort' type of drug and will usually be prescribed when other medications have not worked to manage or treat the symptoms of psychosis (2). Mechanism for action: Clozapine's antipsychotic action is likely mediated through a combination of antogistic effects at D2 receptors in the mesolimbic pathway and 5-HT2A receptors in the frontal cortex. D2 antagonism relieves positive symptoms while 5-HT2A antagonism alleviates negative symptoms (28)

Clozapine is not only unique in the way it is used in treatment, but it is also unique in the adverse side-effects a patient is at risk for (2). Clozapine causes the patient's white blood cell count to decrease making them more septuple to infections (2). Therefore, Clozapine is only recommended for patients that are under close monitoring (29). Other adverse side effects include fever, seizures, constipation, an increased risk of falling due to sedation, hypoglycemia, and an increased mortality rate in the elderly (29). When the patient has concluded their treatment, they will need to be monitored for up to four weeks to monitor the white blood cell count (29).

## RISPERIDONE

Risperidone is a second-generation antipsychotic medication that has been developed to treat irritability in people with autism as well as for the treatment of schizophrenia (30). Risperidone works by attaching itself to the D2 dopamine receptor of the brain and 5-HT2A serotonergic receptors are also impacted (30). With most second-generation medications the chances of experiencing adverse side effects is more rare, however that does not mean that a patient is not at risk of adverse side effects (2). Side effects may include weight gain, blurred vision, dry mouth, low libido, akathisia, diabetes, and constipation (2). Addictiveness is not associated with Aripiprazole but with most antipsychotic medications the body does become dependent, and withdrawal needs to be done gradually (31).

## OLANZAPINE

Olanzapine is used in the treatment of manic episodes associated with bipolar disorder and can be used for the treatment of manic episodes associated with schizophrenia (32). Mechanism of action is understood as:

The activity of olanzapine is achieved by the antagonism of multiple neuronal receptors including the dopamine receptor D1, D2, D3 and D4 in the brain, the serotonin receptors 5HT2A, 5HT2C, 5HT3 and 5HT6, the alpha-1 adrenergic receptor, the histamine receptor H1 and multiple muscarinic receptors. As abovementioned, olanzapine presents a wide profile of targets, however, its antagonistic effect towards the dopamine D2 receptor in the mesolimbic pathway is key as it blocks dopamine from having a potential action at the post-synaptic receptor. The binding of olanzapine to the dopamine D2 receptors is easily dissociable and hence, it allows for a certain degree of dopamine neurotransmission. On the other hand, olanzapine acts in the serotonin 5HT2A receptors in the frontal cortex in a similar manner than the reported on dopamine D2 receptors. This determined effect allows for a decrease in adverse effects (33)

Second-generation antipsychotic medication has fewer adverse side effects when compared to the previous generation developed in the mid to late twentieth-century, however, that does not mean that a patient is no-long at risk of developing adverse side effects and a patient will need to watch out for: weight gain, blurred vision, dry mouth, low libido, akathisia, diabetes, and constipation (2). Addictiveness is unlikely, as most antipsychotic medication is developed to be non-addictive (2).

## QUETIAPINE

Quetiapine was initially approved for use by the FDA in 1997 for the treatment of schizophrenia, bipolar disorder, as well as depression and continues to be used today (34).    Mechanism of action:    Although the mechanism of action of quetiapine is not fully understood, several proposed mechanisms exist. In schizophrenia, its actions could occur from the antagonism of dopamine type 2 (D2) and serotonin 2A (5HT2A) receptors. In bipolar depression and major depression, quetiapine's actions may be attributed to the binding of this drug or its metabolite to the norepinephrine transporter. Additional effects of quetiapine, including somnolence, orthostatic hypotension, and anticholinergic effects, may result from the antagonism of H1 receptors, adrenergic α1 receptors, and muscarinic M1 receptors, respectively (34) Quetiapine, like other second-generation medications for psychosis, carries a low risk in the adverse effects department (34). However, when used by youth and adolescents, suicidal tendencies, suicidal thoughts, and suicidal actions are prevalent (34). Secondly, there is an increased risk of mortality in elderly patients (34).

Both generations of antipsychotic medications come with their risk of adverse side effects and symptoms of withdrawal (2). However, new advances in medication and understanding of psychosis has led to the development of second-generation medication that poses a lower rise for adverse side effects and can therefore be safer to take (2).  As stated previously, addiction is not usually associated with these types of medication, however the body can grow dependent on the medication and can cause an unpleasant withdrawal period.

# CHAPTER 6
## ALTERNATIVE USES OF
## ANTIPSYCHOTIC MEDICATIONS

## Anthony Chen

As indicated in previous chapters, antipsychotic medications are most commonly used to treat schizophrenia and other psychotic conditions such as bipolar disorder, psychotic depression, and various types of psychoses. However, due to their unique neurotransmitter blocking properties, several antipsychotic medications are very useful in treating other conditions. In fact, antipsychotic prescriptions are very common prescriptions for children to treat behavioural issues, and for seniors to treat dementia symptoms. However, antipsychotics have various adverse effects and in some cases, are overprescribed. The following chapter will explore the various alternative uses of antipsychotic medications and evaluate the efficacy and risk of such therapies.

### NAUSEA AND VOMITING

Both typical and atypical antipsychotic medications have been used to treat nausea and vomiting in a variety of situations. After typical antipsychotics were developed in the 1950s, they were commonly used in pediatric practice. Specifically, chlorpromazine was used as an antiemetic in children and infants with respiratory diseases. Early studies found that a large portion of children suffering from conditions associated with vomiting had improved conditions after being given 2mg of chlorpromazine per pound of body weight (1). However, these early studies failed to identify potential side effects, stating that the only observed side effect among children and infants was mild drowsiness (1). Nausea and vomiting in adults was also treated with chlorpromazine, sometimes in combination with narcotic medication to enhance effects. Early studies found that patients reported being completely relieved of nausea after taking 25 mg doses of chlorpromazine along with codeine (2). Withstanding, the use of chlorpromazine in such unnecessary

42

treatments has since been amended heavily due to well-documented side effects. As a typical antipsychotic, chlorpromazine can cause many adverse effects including acute parkinsonism, diabetes, weight gain, and hyperprolactinemia. Chlorpromazine can block the action of acetylcholine, a common neurotransmitter, and cause a myriad of associated side effects (3).

While the use of chlorpromazine to regularly treat nausea and vomiting in otherwise healthy children has been significantly reduced, some prospects of chlorpromazine as an antiemetic to treat children receiving chemotherapy have been proposed. One study found that when children undergoing chemotherapy were assigned 30mg of chlorpromazine per meter-cubed of body volume, they tended to have fewer episodes of vomiting, were less fearful, and were less anxious (4). However, hypertension was induced in one patient, and the mentioned risks of chlorpromazine remain (4).

More recently, the atypical antipsychotic drug, olanzapine, has been used as an antiemetic for cancer patients experiencing refractory nausea and vomiting. Olanzapine is a thienobenzodiazepine and blocks the action of several neurotransmitters including dopamine and serotonin. The goal of prescribing a drug like olanzapine is to reduce opioid requirements to control pain and nausea in advanced cancer patients. One study found that olanzapine acted as an effective antiemetic in cancer patients while inducing less renal and hepatic damage and causing fewer cases of seizures in comparison to other antiemetic drugs (5). However, conditions such as diabetes and prolonged QTC have still been associated with this treatment, thus it must be considered carefully (5).

### AUGMENTING AGENT TO ANTIDEPRESSANTS

Atypical antipsychotics have more recently been used in combination with antidepressants to treat patients with major depressive disorder. Many depressed patients do not have very favorable responses to antidepressants by themselves and thus researchers are searching for methods to enhance antidepressant therapy. Meanwhile, antipsychotics have been known to have antidepressant properties over placebos even when given individually (6). Several atypical antidepressants have been used for antidepressant augmentation including aripiprazole, risperidone, olanzapine, and quetiapine.

Several studies measuring the effect of aripiprazole augmented therapy in comparison to antidepressant monotherapy have found a significant difference. These studies used various scales such as the Hamilton Depression Rating Scale (HAM-D), Clinical Global Impressions-Improvement Scale

(CGI-I), and Global Assessment of Function Scale (GAF) to evaluate improvement in depressive symptoms. Patients treated with aripiprazole consistently improved more and at a faster rate than patients treated with antidepressant monotherapy. However, patients receiving aripiprazole experienced side effects such as restlessness, and headaches (7). Studies in which patients were assigned olanzapine augmented therapies produced similar results of faster improvement in depressive symptoms. However, persistent side effects of drowsiness and heavily increased appetite were found (7). Patients assigned Quetiapine also showed similar improvements in depressive recovery with similar symptoms of sedation, and weight gain (7). Finally, patients treated with risperidone did improve at a faster rate and also held on longer before relapse when compared to a placebo (7).

Generally, in a meta-analysis of 16 trials with antipsychotic augmentation, the augmented therapy was found to be significantly more effective in inducing responses and remission. It was also found that the different antipsychotic drugs: aripiprazole, risperidone, olanzapine, and quetiapine, had similar efficacies (8). The meta-analysis also suggests that atypical antipsychotics have the strongest evidence in being effective in comparison to other augmenting agents such as lithium and buspirone (8). For these reasons, antipsychotic enhanced treatment of depression is becoming a more common strategy in treating nonpsychotic depression.

## Neurodevelopmental Disorders (ASD, ID, ADHD)

Neurodevelopmental disorders including autism spectrum disorder (ASD), and attention-deficit/hyperactivity disorder (ADHD). These disorders frequently cause misconduct and irritability which can put children at risk to harm themselves or to harm others.

In patients with ASD, both risperidone and aripiprazole are used to treat irritability. A meta-analysis of the effects of risperidone found that 5 to 17 year old ASD patients treated with risperidone experienced significantly greater reductions in irritability in 6 to 8 weeks compared to patients given a placebo. However, adverse symptoms such as drowsiness, respiratory tract infections, and weight gain were also observed in patients given risperidone (9). Additionally, in studies where the therapy is discontinued, patients in the risperidone groups showed significantly higher rates of relapse in irritability in comparison to patients in the placebo groups (9). A meta-analysis of the effects of aripiprazole also demonstrated a significant reduction in irritability in ASD patients between 6 and 17 after 8 weeks when they were treated with aripiprazole versus a placebo. Sedation, drooling and tremors were likely to occur in patients treated with aripiprazole, although weight gain was not significantly different (9). Surprisingly, patients who were treated with aripiprazole showed lower likelihood of relapse and longer periods before relapse in comparison to patients given a placebo (9). Generally, while there is evidence supporting the short-term effectiveness of risperidone and aripiprazole in treating irritability in ASD patients, these drugs should be considered a short-term solution, while psychosocial therapy should be used in the long term.

ASD tends to frequently overlap with ADHD, and patients with both disorders tend to suffer more severe social impairment. In a recent study, patients with both ASD and ADHD were treated with risperidone and aripiprazole in order to reduce the symptoms of ADHD (inattention and hyperactivity). It was found that after 24 weeks both aripiprazole and risperidone induced significant improvements in ADHD symptoms according to the ADHD Rating Scale. Some adverse symptoms were found including increased appetite, weight gain, and drowsiness. Nonetheless, these antipsychotics offer an effective alternative pathway to treat ADHD symptoms to nonresponders of standard medications (10).

### Aggressive Youth

Even in individuals who do not suffer from a neurodevelopmental disorder, atypical antipsychotics are sometimes used to treat aggressive behaviour. There is a growing trend of increased antipsychotic prescriptions for children and adolescents within the past two decades, and 77% of children treated with atypical antipsychotics do not have a psychotic disorder (11). Typical antipsychotics were used in the past to treat aggression, with studies showing that haloperidol performed better than lithium and a placebo in reducing childhood aggression (12). However, long-term treatment using typical psychotics causes dyskinesia and can sometimes result in fatal cases of neuroleptic malignant syndrome. For these reasons, the use of typical antipsychotics has been greatly replaced by the use of atypical antipsychotics to treat aggression. Atypical antipsychotics used to treat aggression include olanzapine, clozapine, quetiapine, ziprasidone, and risperidone.

Similar to the use of these drugs to treat behavioural issues in patients with neurodevelopmental disorders, atypical antipsychotics are generally effective in improving behavioural measures in youths. Risperidone was found to produce results better than placebos in only one week of treatment and olanzapine is associated with reductions in self-harm and property damage. While clozapine, quetiapine, and ziprasidone are still widely used in hospitals and residential treatment centers, there is actually very little literature evidence of their effectiveness (12). However, with all these drugs there remains significant safety concerns. As mentioned, weight gain, diabetes, drug-induced movement disorders including dyskinesias, and cardiovascular irregularities associated with atypical antipsychotic use is well documented (12). In most cases, patient treatment should be centered around psychosocial therapy rather than antipsychotics, and research comparing the efficacy of antipsychotics and other classes of drugs to reduce aggression should be pursued (12).

Unfortunately, in a study where children in residential treatment centers were monitored for aggression and treatment, it was found that antipsychotics are frequently over-prescribed. Around 40 to 60% of youth with infrequent or non-aggressive behaviour were treated with antipsychotics during a year of monitoring. Additionally, no reduction in dose over time was observed in youths who stopped showing aggressive behaviour (11). This demonstrates improper handling of antipsychotic prescriptions and the need for reform.

## TIC DISORDER

Patients with Tourette syndrome have motor and vocal tics which can be greatly reduced using antipsychotic drugs. Two antipsychotics are currently approved for tic treatment by the FDA: haloperidol and pimozide. Meta-analysis on the effects of these antipsychotics concluded that they were significantly more effective at reducing tics in comparison to placebos. The effects of different antipsychotics like haloperidol, pimozide, risperidone, and ziprasidone were very similar with no significant differences in efficacy (13). However, these drugs differ in side effects, as mentioned previously, and are not recommended as the first method of treatment for patients with Tourettes (13). Haloperidol is associated with even stronger adverse effects than other typical antipsychotics and pimozide has a strong cardiac risk profile. Even the trials that gave haloperidol and pimozide FDA approval are considerably dated and require re-evaluation (14). While generally recognized as the most effective method of reducing tics, research into alternatives such as alpha-2 agonists has shown similar efficacy in reducing tics in patients who also had ADHD (13). For these reasons, it is not advised to hold off prescribing antipsychotics for Tourettes syndrome until the severity warrants it.

Patients with generalized anxiety disorder are sometimes prescribed atypical antipsychotic drugs by general practitioners even though none of these drugs are approved for the treatment of anxiety. While clinical research into the benefits and risks of this treatment is limited, the existing studies are very promising. Atypical drugs like risperidone, olanzapine, aripiprazole, ziprasidone, and quetiapine have been used to treat anxiety with considerable effectiveness as. A meta-analysis of the efficacy of atypical antipsychotics found that these drugs tended to be effective versus a placebo in both adjunctive therapies with traditional treatments and monotherapies. Rates of remission between adjunctive and monotherapies tended to be similar. However, it was found that only 50% of the patients tolerate the side effects of these drugs (15). Fortunately, the use of low doses of quetiapine (50mg/day) was found to be sufficient in decreasing anxiety symptoms and thus it may be used to develop more tolerable therapies (15). The largest advantage of antipsychotic treatment is that it acts as an alternative to benzodiazepines which produces similar results without leading to withdrawal and addiction. This being the case, antipsychotics should still serve as an alternative to the safer traditional therapies such as cognitive-behavioral therapies and selective serotonin reuptake inhibitors (15).

In practice, an increasing number of prescriptions for antipsychotics are being given to patients with anxiety disorders with quetiapine and aripiprazole as the most popular prescriptions. In a study of drug treatments, 53.6% of inpatients and 16.6% of outpatients with nonpsychotic anxiety disorders were prescribed antipsychotic medication (16). Most patients find antipsychotic medication to be tolerable, and it is currently a great alternative for nonresponders of first-line therapies.

## DEMENTIA

Patients with Alzheimer's disease and other forms of dementia are regularly treated with atypical antipsychotic drugs to reduce symptoms such as delusions, aggression, and agitation. Drugs frequently used in the treatment of dementia include aripiprazole, olanzapine, quetiapine, and risperidone. Meta-analysis of studies on the efficacy of these drugs shows that they are inconsistent in relieving dementia symptoms and sometimes do not outperform placebos. Aripiprazole and risperidone were found to be more effective than olanzapine and quetiapine, but with all drugs, positive responses were rarely seen in outpatients and patients with less severe dementia (17). Additionally, several adverse events occurred in a large number of patients, including urinary tract infections and incontinence (17). In practice, antipsychotic medication should only be used for dementia patients with serious behavioural problems and should be discontinued if improvements are not seen within 10 to 12 weeks.

Moreover, treating dementia symptoms with antipsychotics is associated with an increased rate of mortality. In a study that compared the relative risk of mortality between different antipsychotics, haloperidol prescriptions resulted in the highest rate of mortality followed by risperidone and olanzapine (18). Considering all of this, it is concerning that a quarter of dementia patients in the UK are prescribed antipsychotics in any given year. A good deal of judgement and consideration by patients, their families, and practitioners should be used before the prescription of such drugs to treat dementia (19)

## INSOMNIA

Atypical antipsychotic drugs such as quetiapine are commonly used to treat insomnia even though there is limited literature evidence for its efficacy. Yet, as previously discussed, quetiapine and other atypical antipsychotics are associated with a myriad of adverse side effects. One study, in which patients were assigned quetiapine or a placebo for primary insomnia, found no significant difference in mean sleep time between the groups. Sleep latency and patient satisfaction with their sleep also remained similar between the groups (20). The lack of evidence in this field combined with the well documented adverse effects of the medication suggest that quetiapine and other atypical antipsychotic drugs should not be prescribed for the treatment of insomnia (20)

## DIGESTIVE PROBLEMS

Metoclopramide is similar to other typical antipsychotics but it has, in comparison, weaker antipsychotic properties. Metoclopramide was instead used to stimulate gut motility and reduce vomiting (21). However, due to the adverse effects of typical antipsychotics these practices are not used regularly today. There are, nevertheless , instances of treating diabetic gastroparesis, a condition where the stomach does not contract normally, with metoclopramide. In several studies, patients treated with metoclopramide improved their digestion significantly in comparison to patients given a placebo (22). Generally, metoclopramide is accepted as an effective short-term treatment of gastroparesis even though there is no evidence of long-term benefits (22).

Due to a lack of medications available to treat gastroparesis, metoclopramide is still used as first-line therapy today.

## CONCLUSION

Typical and atypical antipsychotics are effective in treating a variety of conditions. For certain purposes such as tic reduction, the enhancement of antidepressants, and diabetic gastroparesis, antipsychotics are significantly more effective than alternative therapies. In other areas, antipsychotics should be reserved for non-responders of existing first-line therapies due to their high risk profile. Finally, there are some conditions such as dementia and primary insomnia where evidence of antipsychotic efficacy is lacking yet prescriptions are still widespread. Patients and their caretakers should always remember that antipsychotics are physiology altering drugs that should only be prescribed after considering every aspect of their situation,

# CHAPTER 7
## TYPICAL VS. ATYPICAL MECHANISMS OF ACTION?

### John Christy Johnson

Introduction Antipsychotics are often categorized into typical (first-genera-tion) and atypical (second-generation). Both are similar in their mechanisms of action in that they block the D2 Dopamine receptors in the brain and thereby inhibit dopaminergic transmission. However, these therapeutics also have their unique effects on the nervous system and the body as a whole that both healthcare professionals and patients should be aware of prior to starting a course.

It cannot be understated that even today, the mechanism for schizophrenia and other psychiatric conditions that require the use of antipsychotics is not well understood. As such, the content provided during this section should be taken with a grain of salt. Several hypotheses and conjectures have been put forward in this section which ought to be read within the context of the cur-rent time of writing. New, more recent research is constantly being conduct-ed and published and the advances in the field ensure it is continually evolv-ing. At the same time, however, large-scale randomized clinical trials are necessary to validate and provide high- quality evidence for the use of both typical and atypical antipsychotic agents in patients requiring treatment.

Typical drugs are dopamine receptor antagonists including phenothiazines, butyrophenones, thioxanthenes, dibenzoxazepines, dihydroindoles, and diphenylbutylpiperidines. Whereas, atypical drugs are serotonin-dopamine antagonists and include risperidone, olanzapine, quetiapine, ziprasidone, aripiprazole, paliperidone, asenapine, lurasidone, iloperidone, cariprazine, brexpiprazole, and clozapine. For the purposes of this chapter, we will focus on a general mechanism of action for typical/atypical antipsychotics and broader drug classes in particular. [1]

Dopamine Receptor pharmacology Prior to examining the differences between the typical and atypical antipsychotics, it may be useful to have a preliminary understanding of the way these drugs are similar. Both of these therapeutics work extensively on the dopaminergic systems of our body. Dopaminergic systems exist in the central and peripheral nervous systems. In fact, dopamine neurotransmitters and receptors have been identified in various organ systems outside the brain, such as the spinal cord, nerves that supply the heart, and even the gut (in the enteric nervous system).

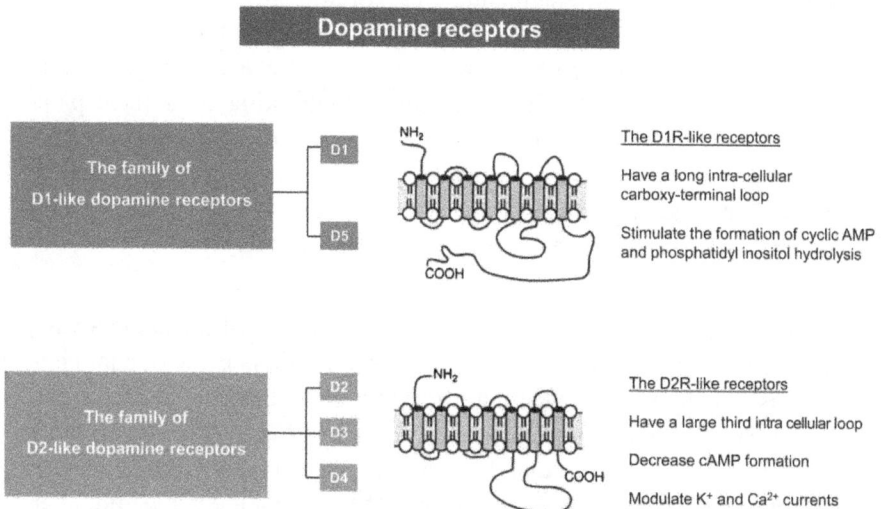

Figure 1: Classification of Dopamine Receptors Function and Structure [2]

There are two broad categories of dopamine receptors - the D1 group (composed of D1 and D5 dopamine receptors) and the D2 group (composed of D2, D3, and D4 dopamine receptors). The receptor families both belong to a class of G-protein coupled receptors, which have a characteristic 7 transmembrane domains. Interestingly, these receptor families have distinct second messenger systems which promote subsequent processes in the cell. [2]

As shown in Figure 1, the receptors are located in the cell membrane and have an amino (-NH2) terminus outside the cell membrane and a carboxy (-COOH) terminus inside the cell. The D1 family of receptors differs from the D2 family of receptors structurally in that it has a long intracellular carboxy-terminal loop of amino acids which make up the protein receptor while the D2 family of receptors have a large third intracellular loop. Functionally, the D1 family of receptors differs from the D2 family of receptors in that it stimulates the formation of cyclic AMP second messengers while the D2 family of receptors decreases the production of cyclic AMP. In doing so, the D2 family of receptors, which includes the D2 dopamine receptors that antipsychotics target, work to modulate cellular ion currents, particularly of K+ and Ca++.

## MECHANISM OF SCHIZOPHRENIA AND OTHER PSYCHIATRIC CONDITIONS

Brain D2 receptors in particular can be found in the highest concentrations in the caudate, putamen (basal ganglia), substantia nigra, nucleus accumbens, and the ventral tegmental area. Additionally, there are thought to be four tracts that dopaminergic transmission is thought to play a role in. These are the mesolimbic pathway, mesocortical pathway, the nigrostriatal pathway, and the tuberoinfundibular pathway. In thinking about these pathways, executive functioning deficits and other cognitive side effects have been linked with mesocortical pathways. Extrapyramidal effects are mediated by the nigrostriatal pathway (discussed in detail later) and raise prolactin levels which can have variable effects on the endocrine systems.

In the clinical context, one of the most popular theories of the pathophysiology of schizophrenia and other psychiatric conditions is the dopamine hypothesis. The hypothesis postulates mesolimbic pathway hyperactivity is the cause of the positive symptoms of schizophrenia. Positive symptoms include hallucinations, paranoia, disorganized speech, and movement disorders among others. There is also evidence for this from the way stimulants such as cocaine can increase dopamine activity in the mesolimbic pathway and how paranoia is something long-term stimulant abusers can often experience. As such, one of the mechanisms thought to be critical in reducing or eliminating positive symptoms is the D2 dopamine receptor blockage.

In its revision, the hypothesis was revised to include another potential pathophysiological mechanism for schizophrenia and other psychiatric conditions. The revised dopamine hypothesis posits that dopamine deficiency in the mesocortical pathway and lack of adequate stimulation of D1 receptors in the prefrontal cortex may be responsible for the negative or cognitive symptoms of schizophrenia. Negative symptoms include blunted affect, lack or poverty of speech and thought, apathy, anhedonia, reduced social drive, loss of motivation, lack of social interest, and inattention to social or cognitive input.

This poses a challenge therapeutically for drug designers as the ideal drug would selectively have to decrease dopamine in the mesolimbic pathway to alleviate positive symptoms and increase dopamine in the mesocortical pathway to treat negative and cognitive symptoms.

The last hypothesis we consider here is the glutamate hypothesis. While this is not as relevant for our discussion on typical and atypical antipsychotic drugs, it should be noted that our current drug strategies focus on acting downstream of the critical neurotransmitter abnormality and future drug development should focus on manipulating upstream factors. Blockade of the NMDA glutamate receptor complex has previously been described to mimic schizophrenia and psychosis in terms of both positive and negative symptoms, making it an interesting target for future therapeutic targeting and intervention.

## TYPICAL ANTIPSYCHOTIC DRUGS

These drugs are primarily used to treat schizophrenia and related psychotic disorders. They are also still used despite the availability of atypical antipsychotics due to their inexpensiveness. Based on our current understanding, typical antipsychotic drugs have their antipsychotic effects predominantly by one mechanism - by antagonizing the D2 dopamine receptors. Other effects include the antagonism of M1 muscarinic receptors, H1 histaminergic receptors, and alpha-1 adrenergic receptors, among others.

History: In 1951, the first reported use of typical antipsychotic phenothiazines was documented. Phenothiazines were developed for their antihistaminergic properties to treat inflammation and allergies. Similarly, another typical antipsychotic chlorpromazine was administered for its potential anesthetic effects during surgery. Shortly thereafter, the use of both these drugs were extended to the treatment of psychiatric patients, and by a stroke of luck, their antipsychotic activity was discovered. [3]

Science: The blockade of D2 receptors in the brains has been examined using PET scans to suggest that for some antipsychotic drugs, one may see a loss of efficacy at higher doses. For example, symptoms of OCD have been suggested for higher doses >65% dopamine D2/3/4 occupancy of the atypical antipsychotic clozapine. However, typical antipsychotic drugs particularly haloperidol have been associated with a high potency with >78% dopamine D2/3/4. The problem with higher potency is that one is more likely to get extrapyramidal side effects.

Limitations: Extrapyramidal symptoms can broadly be thought of as motor disorders and are common complications of typical antipsychotics. Mechanistically, these can be attributed to the role of high concentration of dopamine D2 receptors in the caudate and putamen. These are brain regions which are associated with fluid and concerted movement and coordination.

As such, it may not be surprising to learn that symptoms can include dystonia, a muscle problem that causes continuous spasms and muscle contractions. There could also be akathisia, a condition which can manifest as motor restlessness. Similarly, parkinsonism or Parkinson syndrome-like characteristic symptoms can also be seen such as rigidity, slow movement, tremor, and jerky, irregular motion (tardive dyskinesia). Note that other adverse systemic effects in other parts of the body also exist but are not discussed as atypical antipsychotics have similar and/or comparatively negligible effects.

### SEROTONIN RECEPTOR PHARMACOLOGY

Atypical antipsychotics have effects on various classes of serotonin receptors, so it would be worthwhile to review some of the basic pharmacological characteristics of the serotonin 5-HT receptor. In the brain, serotonergic pathways are found in the midbrain raphe nuclei and project upwards into higher centers of the brain and down the spinal cord. Besides the diffuse concentration of serotonin in the brain, serotonin also exists in the gut, blood, among others. There are at least 15 different types of serotonin receptor classes. For our purposes, we will be considering 5-HT1A and 5-HT2A receptors.

5-HT1A, similar to dopamine D2 receptors, uses an inhibitory G-protein coupled receptor pathway. It works by negatively coupling to second messenger adenylyl cyclase and is positively coupled to G protein-coupled inwardly-rectifying potassium channels which control the potassium currents. It will also induce neuronal inhibition as well as presynaptic inhibition.

5-HT2A, on the other hand, employs a completely different G-protein coupled receptor mechanism. Activation of the receptor triggers a cascade of enzymatic changes that stems from the activation of beta-type phospholipase C enzymes, eventually leading to the phosphorylation of cellular targets that promote neuronal excitation and smooth muscle contraction.

### ATYPICAL ANTIPSYCHOTIC DRUGS

Atypical antipsychotic drugs have lower potency and generally have more histaminergic action and are more sedating. This class also has generally less D2 blocking potency or affinity for receptors but has roughly equal efficacy or effect for treating positive symptoms of schizophrenia and other psychoses. One of the advantages of atypical antipsychotic medications is the reduction of extrapyramidal symptoms and sometimes is the defining feature for atypical antipsychotics. Based on our current understanding, there are three mechanisms of action by which atypical antipsychotics are hypothesized to exert their antipsychotic effects - 5-HT2A Serotonin receptor/D2 dopamine receptor antagonism, rapid D2 dissociation, and 5-HT1A Serotonin receptor agonism.

With 5-HT2A Serotonin receptor/D2 dopamine receptor antagonism, the theory is that the serotonin-dopamine balances play a role in ameliorating the symptoms of psychosis. Keeping in mind the mechanistic action of serotonin to promote neuromuscular excitation, inhibiting serotonergic actions may prevent some of the positive symptoms seen in schizophrenia. However, in the bigger picture, 5-HT2A receptors can easily be blocked at the lower dosages of most atypical antipsychotic drugs and could just as likely be a side effect of lower-potency configurations of the drugs. This means that D2 dopamine receptor blockade remains the primary mode of action, regardless of whether 5-HT2A receptor antagonism is present. [4]

It has been shown that typical antipsychotics like haloperidol bind more tightly than dopamine itself to the dopamine D2 receptor, with experimentally-derived dissociation constants that are much lower than that for dopamine. One important hypothesis for this has been the 'hit and run' described by Stahl in 2001. [5]

The hit and run mechanism action is hypothesized to work due to the rapid D2 dissociation. In comparison to the conventional antipsychotic, the atypical antipsychotic will attach to or 'hit' the D2 receptor for a shorter period of time before dissociation or 'run'. This means that there is less potency for the atypical antipsychotic. The advantages of this include fewer spikes in prolactin levels,cognitive impairment, and extrapyramidal symptoms. There is also another theory that builds off this one that is used to predict which antipsychotic agents will or will not produce adverse effects called the 'fast-off D2 theory' which suggests a correlation between the dissociation of the antipsychotic with the effectiveness of the treatment. [4]

The final mechanism suggests that atypical antipsychotics have some 5-HT1A stimulatory effects. Noting its similarity of mechanism to D2 receptor antagonism, it is easy to conjecture that promoting the inhibitory serotonergic effects through agonism can mimic the inhibitory dopaminergic effects promoted by antagonism. That being said, this is not a significant mechanism of action and if it does exist, it is most likely to merely complement the D2 receptor antagonism.

History: Between 1954 and 1975, 40 antipsychotic drugs were introduced throughout the world with the most well-known being the typical antipsychotic haloperidol. The problem with this potent antipsychotic was its extrapyramidal symptoms which rendered patients who were on the drug into parkinsonian states. Thereafter, there was a hiatus in the development of antipsychotics until the re-introduction of clozapine in the US in 1990 began the era of atypical antipsychotics. [3]

Science: In 2005, the Clinical Antipsychotic Trials of Intervention Effectiveness (CATIE) project sponsored by the National Institute of Mental Health was designed to compare the typical antipsychotic perphenazine to several atypical antipsychotics [6]. CATIE results were significant in that they established these second-generation antipsychotics as a much more effective and preferable clinical option than typical antipsychotics. However, while olanzapine was deemed to be the most effective in the CATIE trial, there were substantive metabolic complications associated with olanzapine.

Limitations: Some of the complications of atypical antipsychotics included the worsening baseline metabolic problems it created. Several reports compound the negative metabolic picture painted by atypicals including Increased dyslipidemia risk, increased diabetes mellitus risk, which can happen in one week with clozapine, and insulin resistance can occur as early as 6 weeks. [7] Several theories exist for these effects including increased intake, decreased activity, slow metabolism, or a combination of these. There is also a direct correlation between H1 binding affinity and the degree of weight gain associated with the antipsychotic drug.

### CLOSING THOUGHTS

Both typical and atypical antipsychotics have undergone periods of use and refinement. Typical antipsychotic medications were potent, effective, and sometimes led to extrapyramidal symptoms due to their effects on the D2 dopamine receptor while atypicals addressed this problem to leave new metabolic concerns with its use. One of the biggest problems associated with these medications is that the medical condition itself appears to have its own uncertainties. Even today, schizophrenia and psychosis are poorly understood with many hypotheses and conjectures around their mechanism of action.

Here, we have reviewed the basic pharmacological mechanisms of dopaminergic and serotonergic receptors and put them in the context of these antipsychotics and the clinical implications for patients with schizophrenia and psychosis. Taken collectively, in addition to the D2 blocking effects, atypical antipsychotic drugs also have a couple of other mechanisms of action. This includes the ability for atypical antipsychotic agents to act as a 5-HT2A Serotonin receptor antagonist and a 5-HT1A serotonin receptor agonist. These mechanistic features in conjunction with the drugs' effects on D2 receptors make it a much more versatile drug class.

Looking towards the future, further developments are being conducted even today to prevent some of the adverse side effects associated with these drugs. Pharmaceuticals have had developments in marketing campaigns as well with first, second, and now third generations of antipsychotics. The hope is that these next generations of these compounds can reduce the severity of extrapyramidal symptoms, metabolic complications, and other systemic issues that were not discussed in this chapter. Nevertheless, the marketing should not underscore the importance of the constant need for more rigorous research through randomized clinical trials.

# CHAPTER 8
## PSYCHOSOCIAL TREATMENTS THAT ARE USED IN CONJUNCTION WITH ANTIPSYCHOTICS

### Avery Kennedy

There are currently many psychosocial treatment methods being used with medication for the treatment of psychosis, and many more being studied and created as time goes on. They are all diagnosis specific and many different theories exist for how to approach psychosocial treatment and what to target. This chapter will examine some of the approaches taken to treating schizophrenia, how treatment differs in older patients and investigate studies in the extremely under researched category of youth demonstrating self-injurious thoughts and behaviours.

Overtime psychologists have concluded that medication is not sufficient for the treatment and recovery of schizophrenia. Therefore, the use of psychosocial treatment is gaining traction and being researched more and more. In their study, Kern et al. discuss four of the most well established and commonly researched methods of psychosocial treatments for Schizophrenia. This chapter with cover three:" Social Skills Training, Cognitive Behavioural Therapy, and Social Cognition Training.[3]

According to Kern et al., Social Skills Training is the most researched method and has the longest history. Treatment can be done in groups or individually and has evolved to include outpatients in society, not just hospitalized patients. This sort of training targets social skills and is based on the Social Learning Theory. A movement in the 1960s and 70s started to bring social learning principles into the psychiatry space. These principles are useful in treating schizophrenia for a few reasons. Patients often exhibit inappropriate, excessive or deficient behaviours which can be measured and are therefore, easier to study. These behaviours acted as barriers to patients adapting to the social world and achieving their goals. Humans are fundamentally social and their environment shapes their behaviour, which is a strong indication that the Social Skills Training would have an effect. These skills can also be taught to people experiencing more severe symptoms associated with schizophrenia such as hallucinations and delusions. Due to these findings, social skills training is now widely used.[3]

However, it can be difficult to measure the effectiveness of this training, which has led to some mixed results in studies that range from very positive to much more doubtful conclusions. One reason could be that the parameters being measured are symptoms and relapses, which has a questionable connection to social skills as many factors can contribute to a relapse. There are also questions about the potential for generalization these treatments offer. It is unclear whether the skills learned in trial are able to be effectively utilized in a non-clinical setting. Despite these challenges, there is some evidence that has been studied more recently which indicates a rate of effectiveness with these sort of trials and have indicated that they have the potential to have wider effects in the recovery and social skills of patients with schizophrenia. Therefore, , Kern et al. highlight the importance of "planning generalization" so the skills learned benefit the recipients of treatment in society.[3]

Kern et al. then move on to Cognitive Behavioural Therapy (CBT), which targets improvement of social skills, quality of life, and cognitive impairments to improve social and work functioning. It has been shown that the symptoms of schizophrenia contribute to lower social engagement and that treatment can have a positive impact on social engagement of the patient. CBT may sound similar to Social Skills Training but it takes a different approach on account of a different base theory. "CBT is based on the Cognitive Model of Psychopathology,"[3] meaning that biological factors are the initial cause of illness but that faulty cognitive appraisal, or the faulty interpretation of events, results in the full illness. The theory therefore targets this faulty perception for treatment. With psychoses, this theory sees medication as necessary but part of a larger treatment needed. Several manuals with slight differences in this approach to treatment but all include "engagement and assessment; coping enhancement; developing a shared understanding of the experience of psychosis; (…) working on delusions and hallucinations; (…) addressing mood and negative self evaluations; and managing the risk of relapse."[3]

Social Cognition Training targets the "mental operations underlying social interactions" the impairment of which, indicated "poor functional outcome in schizophrenia."[3] Social cognitive impairment can include difficulty "perceiving, interpreting, and generating responses to the intentions, dispositions, and emotions of others."[3] Social cognition also appears to have a strong connection with functional outcome and is therefore a good target for treatment. Social cognition training is the newest form of treatment out of the three explored here but it is already showing promising signs in longer term and targeted studies. It has shown improvement in social cognition processes and perception in patients with schizophrenia, which "have been linked to successful social functioning."[3] It seems as though this field of research could hold some promising treatments in this future.[3]

According to Kern et al., one orientation that is widely recognized across all methods of treatment is that patients are "more than the sum of their symptoms."[3] This can allow for more goal-oriented therapy with patients working to improve their skills in order to achieve certain goals such as being employed. It also allows patients to have a sense of self beyond their symptoms. Because of this "all formal definitions of recovery include criteria to address symptom stability or freedom from psychiatric hospitalization," and include "normalization of social and work/school functioning."[3] There is very little research explicitly targeting this definition of recovery for a variety of reasons, including length of follow ups and the many factors that contribute to recovery, which make it difficult to narrow it down to one or two factors of treatment. Kern et al. state that more should be done in this field of research to help improve psychosocial treatment.[3]

After discussing some treatment approaches for schizophrenia, one can see there are several methods that hold promising results. However, how do the strategies change when dealing with a different set of the population? In their paper, Jeste and Maglione discuss the challenges and opportunities present when treating older patients with schizophrenia. An important thing to note before diving into this discussion is that Jeste and Maglione's definition of older as it relates to schizophrenia is perhaps slightly different than that of the general population. They say that because patients with schizophrenia are "reported to have accelerated physical aging," and a lifespan that is around 20 years shorter than average; a person with schizophrenia in their 40s can be compared to a member of the general population in their 60s. Older schizophrenia patients also have less severe positive symptoms of schizophrenia and are more often hospitalized because of physical problems instead of relapse.[2]

The first major difference between the treatment of an older patient and a younger one is caused by the natural way that schizophrenia develops overtime. In adults with late-onset schizophrenia, aging has been "associated with improved psychological function, less substance use, decreased psychotic symptoms, reduced risk of psychiatric hospitalization, and improved mental health-related quality of life."[2] Some have a "sustained remission of illness,"[2] which means their symptoms are either reduced or completely gone. Jeste and Maglione have also found that in this category, patients can be taken completely off antipsychotic medication or have their doses reduced below 50%.[2]

There is an increased risk of side effects from antipsychotic medication in this population and they say that a minority of patients can be phased off antipsychotics. They also highlight various psychosocial treatment plans that could help the functioning of patients which includes Social Skills Training. They cite a few studies that used various combinations of CBT, Social Skills Training and others which all resulted in improved social functioning. They also mention the potential benefit of mobile devices to deliver treatment to patients in the community.[2]

In general, Jeste and Maglione emphasise the importance of lowering doses to the absolute minimum, the close monitoring of patients during this process and the need for psychosocial therapy as an accompaniment. As is common in literature on this subject, they illustrate the gaps in research that must be filled in order to advance treatment efficacy and develop new treatment strategies. They also highlight that more research needs to be done to better understand the difference between women and men with schizophrenia.[2]

Now we will discuss psychosocial treatment methods and research in another field. The article by Glen et al. tackles psychosocial treatment research for youth with self-injurious thoughts and behaviours (SITB) which are usually divided into suicidal and non-suicidal behaviours and thoughts. Although these categories are separate, research does indicate there is a "significant risk factor for suicidal behaviour"[1] when people demonstrate non-suicidal behaviours, which include non-suicidal self-injury and suicide threats. "In the United States, suicide is third leading cause of death in youth"[1] Each year around 16% adolescents consider suicide, 13% make a plan, and 8% attempt suicide. Currently in US, "most suicidal adolescents have received some form of mental health treatment" and the "rate of treatment for suicidal behaviour as increased"[1] According to Glen et al. these behaviours have not fallen despite these facts. This may indicate that the treatment options and approach of this field needs to be more effective..

In their literature review, studies were separated into categories of family involvement. Family was categorized as "treatments where family was the primary focus of the intervention," Individual + Family was categorized as "interventions that focused on individual skills training" and used family therapy as part of treatment, and Individual treatments focused on adolescents with optional or no family sessions.[1]

Self-injurious thoughts and behaviours (SITB) and other maladaptive behaviours could come from "distorted thinking patterns and deficits in specific skills,"[1] such as regulating emotions and problem solving. Therefore, CBT has been investigated with the aim to reduce SITBs by modifying cognitive distortions and strengthening communication, problem solving, and coping skills. Out of the CBT-individual studies they investigated, one had an 36% drop out rate and no control group. It was also a very small study. These factors mean that despite an indication of reduction in Deliberate self-harm (DSH) maintained at a three-month follow up, more research is needed to be done in order to indicate proof. The other study indicated "individual CBT is not superior to supportive therapy."[1] The CBT-individual + CBT-family treatment included individual and family sessions. One study with a very small sample size found reduction in suicidal idealation (SI) but not substance abuse (SA) (third of group attempted suicide during treatment), no comparison group therefore conclusions are difficult to prove and still very tentative. A larger study with a sample of over 100 was focused specifically on treatment for adolescents who had attempted suicide and experienced major depression. They compared CBT-SP, medication, and both combined but found no difference between groups in rates of suicide, attempted suicide, preparatory acts demonstrating suicidal behaviour or suicidal thoughts. However, it was noted that SE rates were lower in their trial after 6 months when compared with naturalistic studies of patients considered high-risk after hospital discharge.[1] Different circumstances between the studies make it difficult to compare and more studies are needed. The evidence provided in these two trials makes it difficult to draw any certain conclusions.

In the CBT-individual + CBT-family + Parent Training trials, one created ingrained CBT (I-CBT) by combining the three aspects of the previous trials discussed in this paper and compared I-CBT to enhanced typical treatment. Rates of SI decreased in both and SA decreased significantly more in I-CBT along with a reduction in suicidal behaviour, and less drug and alcohol use. More people stayed through to the end of this study than in the other studies discussed so far in this chapter. Due to these factors, this intervention has been classified as Level 2: probably efficacious although it is important to note that this study only included adolescents with reported substance use disorders and therefore should be replicated in more diverse populations of suicidal adolescents.[1]

Another study done by Rudd and colleagues studies CBT - Group therapy in adolescents and young adults ages 15-24 in "daily psychoeducation and skills training groups for 2 weeks."[1] There was a reduction in SI but it did not have more efficacy than standard treatment. Therefore, it was rated "Level 4: experimental" by Glen et al. because of failure to demonstrate more efficacy.

Dialectical Behaviour Therapy (DBT) is "one of the first treatments to specifically target SITBs"[1] It was intended for adult female patients with borderline personality disorder and adapted for adolescents even without a borderline diagnosis. It is meant to teach patients to "regulate their emotional and interpersonal difficulties in adaptive ways."[1] This way they will not turn to SITBs. Generally, the design for this treatment is individual therapy, group skills training, and phone skills coaching. Several studies done with some variation of this design showed reduction in SITBs but with no control group, it is difficult to definitively prove this was a result of the trial. They also mostly included women with BPD and more research is needed to determine whether these treatments are effective in more diverse clinical applications. When investigating other studies there were similarly inconclusive results and "no published studies to date have found that DBT is superior to an active treatment control."[1] Therefore Glen et al. state that studies of longer duration are needed and rate this method as "Level 4: experimental"[1]

Family Based Therapy (FBT) targets "family functioning"[1] to lower SITBs. There are various categorizations based on the techniques used. They generally fall under the umbrella of "psychoeducation, communication training, and problem solving."[1] Some examples include FBT-Attachment, which focuses on improving relationships of the family. This showed significant reductions in SI which were maintained after treatment, and despite limitations like a high dropout rate, Glen et al. classified this technique as "Level 2: probably efficacious."[1] Another method classified at Level 2 was parent only training, which educated parents about SITBs, "effective parenting and decreasing conflict and stress."[1]

A more long-term study focused on reducing environmental factors was promising and, because it focused mainly on African American youth, it also represented a portion of the population that is very underrepresented in medical research. Some factors like a very high rate of hospitalization mean that the study was ranked as Level 3: possibly efficacious. Other studies have investigated behavioral techniques, interpersonal, authority relationships, and increasing access to support and resources.

Overall, none of these treatments have been certified "Level 1: well-established" to treat SITBs. It is clear that more research needs to be done in order to address the treatment of a very large population of patients in the U.S. In general there is promising research in the field of psychosocial treatment but there is a significant need for more research to be done in order to have the best options available to treat patients alongside antipsychotic medication.

# CHAPTER 9
## SOCIETAL IMPACTS OF ANTIPSYCHOTICS AND THE ACCESSIBILITY AND COMMERCIALIZATION OF ANTIPSYCHOTICS

### Belinda Tam

This chapter will discuss the societal impact of antipsychotics and the accessibility and commercialization of antipsychotics. To understand this chapter thoroughly, let's first reinforce the definition of antipsychotics. Antipsychotics is a type of medication used to treat patients with psychosis, bipolar disorder, and schizophrenia. Psychosis is what occurs when individuals see or hear things that do not match reality (hallucinations) and can be part of disorders such as schizophrenia, personality disorder and bipolar disorder. However, it is possible to have these psychotic symptoms without having any of the conditions listed above. Following will be a quick description of the three main disorders impacted by the use of antipsychotics. Bipolar disorder is based in the brain and "causes changes in a person's mood, energy, and ability to function."(6) Individuals with this disorder can go through phases where they experience different emotional states which tend to occur at specific times. The last major disorder associated with antipsychotic medication is schizophrenia. Schizophrenia is a chronic brain disorder that has similar symptoms to bipolar disorder but includes "disorganized speech, trouble with thinking, and lack of motivation."(6) Antipsychotics are used as medication in either short or long-term treatment of these disorders in order to control the symptoms associated with them including hallucinations, delusions, or mania symptoms (2). With that being said, this medication affects people differently and results in various side effects or generally impacts individuals if taken with other medication.

Going back to the topic of this chapter — how antipsychotics may have societal impacts and the accessibility and commercialization of antipsychotics, it is essential to shed light upon the various types of antipsychotic medications. This will allow for a deeper understanding of societal impacts and commercialization. There are two main types of antipsychotics — typical (first generation) and atypical (second generation). The main difference between the two types is the side effects associated with each type.(1)

When comparing the first-generation antipsychotics with the second-generation ones, the former tends to have more of an impact on movement in comparison to atypical antipsychotics. However, we should think of each antipsychotic medication individually as each person's medication is individually prescribed and the impact that the medication has on an individual may differ. With that being said, finding the right medication for each and every patient is very important. When it comes to commercialization, researchers must first look into the size of the market and if incorporating these ideas into a business, there must also be a system in place for both the people manufacturing the product and for those sending out the product. Having a system in place will help with retaining customer satisfaction and loyalty. Lastly, when thinking about manufacturing the medication for the patient, the company also needs to take into account the relationship they have with the physicians and clearly communicate with them for the benefit of the customer.

Next, it is important to point out that the medication can come in three different forms — tablets, syrup, or injection. In terms of commercialization and accessibility then, antipsychotics coming in different forms will definitely have an impact on commercialization due to the commonality of each form. However, for accessibility, this may be more dependent on other businesses that are also manufacturing medication. Currently, tablets and syrups are more common than injections so prices should be adjusted accordingly. Furthermore, depending on what the physician prescribes, there may be fluctuations in terms of commercialization as doctors may not get as many patients who want/need a certain form. This may lead to companies not having to manufacture as much. It is also important to take into account competitive advantage if some companies are able to offer all three forms while others are not — this makes the company that can offer all three forms more diversified and well-rounded. This may also affect pricing the prescriptions as patients may compare companies for the same prescription.

### ACCESSIBILITY OF ANTIPSYCHOTICS AND THE IMPACT ON SOCIETY

If the accessibility of antipsychotics is made more readily available for individuals, society as a whole would benefit more, especially when the patient is caught in a situation/emergency and does not have time to wait for the medication to be prepared. In terms of research in this area, it is interesting as not much has been done in terms of analysis of a greater population and possibly making generalizations to help the everyday individual. It would also be interesting to see how the everyday individual using their medication is prepared for tough situations on both a short and long-term basis. Another reason why this is significant is due to how the individual would be impacted if they did not have the medication, especially in comparison to other patients with different disorders and many other medications on the market. Especially due to the fact that you cannot buy antipsychotics in a drugstore (because you need a prescription), finding the way to make the medication more accessible for patients and getting the medication into the patient's hands faster may result in a profitable business with more individuals satisfied with their overall lifestyle.

## WHEN PATIENTS WANT TO STOP TAKING ANTIPSYCHOTICS

If patients want to stop taking antipsychotics, it is important to discuss with the doctor as medication is reduced over time. "If you stop taking antipsychotics suddenly it can cause 'rebound psychosis'. This means that the symptoms of your illness return suddenly and you may become unwell again."(1) In terms of this affecting commercialization and accessibility, it will first result in a decrease of profit but it would not necessarily affect the accessibility of antipsychotics because the medication is made for one patient. However, because medication is personalized (made for one person), it will result in the loss of a customer (patient) long-term if the patient decides to go off of the medication resulting in the money not being made back. With that being said, readers will probably be asking why the patient may decide to go off of the medication and that is what we are going to be exploring next. One reason in particular is due to the physician deciding that the patient's overall condition has changed or the medication is affecting the patient due to other medications that the patient is taking alongside their antipsychotic medication. This leads into the discussion of the next topic which includes questioning how antipsychotics affect an individual's condition. Since the medication is prescribed on an individual basis, the interaction between medication in each person will vary. With that being said, it is important for the physician to know that to be cautious in general and for the patient to inform the physician of all the medication that they are taking so that the physician can in turn prescribe the correct antipsychotic for the patient. This also impacts commercialization as if the patient is satisfied they will become a loyal customer and may also refer other patients to the business.

Furthermore, changes to the prescription can also occur in terms of a smaller or larger dosage of the medication. If a business is selling the product based on the form and dosage (amount), sales may decrease and increase respectively depending on how much is sold. If building this into a business, this would be a very interesting area of research to go into when looking into other things including the market size, competitors, profit that other businesses have seen, number of employees to hire, rent, etc.

The patient deciding to go off the medication can also have a societal impact depending on how that individual behaves when they are on medication versus when they are off it. Although no generalizations can be made at this point in time, how individuals behave can definitely affect the relationships they have with other people. To a certain extent, this is dependent on how much medication they are taking and how often but what people say about you and the image that people have of you can impact other areas of that patient's life. For the patient themselves, they may end up having poor adherence to medication in general and possibly have a relapse during maintenance treatment. This may also impact how a business will market itself, especially if there are negative connections formed between patients and the business. From a business standpoint, having people in society view you in a positive light can and may impact the overall performance of your business.

### PATIENT CHARACTERISTICS

Characteristics of each individual can have an influence on how the medication may act on their body and in turn, affect how not only society views them but that medication and the company that creates them. This is especially true for the elderly as they are more likely to have adverse effects for a variety of reasons. In comparison to young adults, the elderly have a lower body mass which includes a high proportion of fat to body water, "and decreased renal and hepatic function." (3) These facts help demonstrate that at any given dose, an elderly person is more sensitive to drug effects and that they are more likely to take several drugs; therefore "increasing the risk of adverse effects secondary to drug interactions."(3)

Other characteristics that may come into play when discussing how the medication may affect the individual are gender and [comorbid] physical illness. Women are generally more likely to develop "hyperprolactinaemia[12] and QTc prolongation when treated with antipsychotics"(3) in comparison to men. In practice though, all of these characteristics may also affect the antipsychotic drug chosen by the physician.

To summarize, although much work has been done on this area of research, more should be done to compare populations and cross-study comparisons of tolerability. This may in turn also help understand how the medication can be made more effective and accessible as well since it would be interesting to see medications made generally for certain groups of people.

## ANTIPSYCHOTICS & ITS IMPACT ON DIFFERENT GROUPS
## (FOCUS ON PREGNANT WOMEN)

As we previously discussed, antipsychotics are mainly used to help patients with psychosis, bipolar disorder, and schizophrenia. If we are to look at the antipsychotic market from a business perspective, it is important to consider who may benefit from using this product. The following section will discuss this topic with a focus and analysis of how pregnant women may also find antipsychotics useful and beneficial to them.

During pregnancy, how often and the amount of antipsychotics used are the major factors involved that will result in the largest impacts on the baby. In Scaffer et al., it was found that women who use antipsychotics long-term were more likely to have schizophrenia or be diagnosed with bipolar disorder themselves. They also tend to have elevated rates of various birth outcomes (across the board) in comparison to unexposed women and those with the greatest antipsychotic exposure have the highest percentages of gestational diabetes and hypertension. This demonstrates some of the various effects that antipsychotics can have on pregnancy. It was also found that women who used antipsychotics, especially during pregnancy tended to have patterns and their associated birth outcomes which reflect the differences between women with the same diagnosis. This resulted in differing treatment plans and various severity levels of different illnesses. Moreover, as stated in Schaffer et al., "this diversity should be considered when developing clinical guidelines and designing safety studies."(5) At this point, it has been proved that antipsychotics mainly have a negative effect on women with pregnancy but for future research, it would be interesting to see how this medication can be beneficial for pregnant women. The researchers from this study also observed that women who used a large amount of their medication on a daily basis had the highest rates of preterm birth and babies diagnosed with neonatal abstinence syndrome, gestational diabetes, and hypertension. It is definitely questionable as to whether this will impact the generations after the baby and become a long-term part of the family's medical history. (That being said, the researchers said that this study is purely descriptive so please keep this in mind when reading.) Going back to pregnant women, it was also found that "[l]ong-term antipsychotic use increases the risk of obesity, metabolic syndrome and weight gain [during] pregnancy, all risk factors for gestational diabetes and other complications."(5) Research may question if this may also be the result of the women using antipsychotics before she was pregnant and if not, how would it impact the child if this were the case? More research has been done on this as a result and women who continue to use antipsychotics throughout pregnancy have a strong correlation with a high level of severity of psychiatric illness. This may be due to the fact that the use of antipsychotics is mainly advised for women who have a high risk of relapse in their disorder which may also result in poor birth outcomes for the child. Since so many things can differ, each woman will have their own treatment plans as well. Some factors that are taken into consideration include the woman's needs, circumstances, benefits and risk of all available options which include psychotherapy, medication, or a combination of the two (4). If the woman is prescribed medication, it should be taken at the lowest possible dosage and she should be aware that if she nurses her child(ren) while taking medication, a small amount of the medication will transfer into breast milk. However, the medication may or may not affect the baby depending on the medication itself and when it is taken. These associated risks should be informed to the woman. Besides the physical healing of the woman though, physicians should also be taking mental health into consideration as women may have depression after the baby is born. In terms of commercialization of antipsychotics based on the facts given by this section, it can be said that we mainly see the use of antipsychotics in the negative view. However, future research may want to look at why this is the case and how it can be used to benefit pregnant women and other groups and/or topics such as alcohol and sex.

# CHAPTER 10
# HOW ARE ANTIPSYCHOTIC MEDICATIONS PORTRAYED IN POPULAR CULTURE AND THE MEDIA? HOW ARE THEY PORTRAYED DIFFERENTLY AROUND THE WORLD?

April Sui

As with the perception of various medical treatments, the representation of antipsychotic medications can have an undeniable influence on the use of such drugs by physicians and patients. This chapter aims to provide an overview of different ways in which antipsychotic medications are portrayed in popular culture through examining primarily English based media. Furthermore, the differences in representation of these medications between varying cultures will be briefly explored.

## ADVERTISING AND COMMERCIALS FOR ANTI-PSYCHOTIC MEDICATIONS

A prominent and vocal exhibition of attitudes towards ant-psychotic drugs would be advertisements that address these products. Some interesting disparities between the representation of antipsychotic drugs in relation to men compared to women can be found after examination of different commercials. A 2004 study of psychotropic drug advertisements in the English language looked at how different demographics were portrayed in adverts from the Canadian Journal of Psychiatry, British Journal of Psychiatry, and the American Journal of Psychiatry (1). Data was collected at three separate time intervals (1981, 1991, and 2001) (1). After testing for statistically significant associations by using chi-square analysis, it was found that 57% of the advertisements in the study depicted women as primary patients (1). Previous studies have also demonstrated discrepancies in the proportions of men and women appearing for certain types of medication commercials. An earlier 1995 study of American medical literature found the female to male ratio for advertisements for antidepressants to be 5:1 in the American Journal of Psychiatry (AJP) and 10:0 in American Family Physician (2).

Additionally, there were evident environmental differences between how the sexes were shown in conjunction to their illnesses and psychotropic drugs. In advertisements featuring men from the 2004 study, medication was shown to target short-term, work-related stresses in association with effective coping strategies (1). Women were portrayed in relation to medication for diffusing emotional symptoms and ineffective coping strategies (1). Moreover, 75% of patients who were shown to be in their homes and/or gardens were women (1). For patients portrayed in work and social situation category surroundings, men comprised 85% and 59% respectively (1).

Despite the prevalence of female representation in advertising for general psychotropic drugs, men were featured significantly more often in advertisements for specifically antipsychotic medications (1). It might be concluded that such drugs are commonly seen as mental illness treatment more targeted towards male patients, in particular those who face difficulty in their jobs or social life due to their illnesses. However, gender discriminatory prescribing has declined as of the early 90s (1,2). While a 1985 National Ambulatory Medical Care Survey discovered that women were nearly twice as likely as men to be prescribed antidepressants and anxiolytics, they were just as likely as men to receive prescriptions for antipsychotic drugs or barbiturates (1,2). Yet, in cases where there was not an appropriate diagnosis, female patients were more likely to receive prescriptions for antidepressants and antipsychotics than male patients (2).

The study also made findings on expressed attitudes regarding the apparent effects of psychotropic drugs such as antipsychotic medication. In 23 of 129 studied advertisements, the changes among patients were depicted using before and after images showing the patients' progress from negative (i.e., sad, crying) to positive (i.e., happy, laughing) or neutral (i.e., without apparent effect) states of being (1). It becomes evident that the advertisements portrayed such medications positively and emphasized their therapeutic efficiency.

Though it is understandable that the drugs would be shown in a primarily positive position with disregard to potential side effects, the stark contrast between the before (e.g., in bed, crying) and after (e.g., exuberant, communing with friends) images of the patients depicted an unrealistic therapeutic progression for the average patient (1). Such representations of the medications' impact could strengthen biases of physicians and pharmaceuticals regarding total drug failure and adverse reactions which are in reality noticeable among psychotropic drugs (1).

## ANTIPSYCHOTIC MEDICATIONS IN TELEVISION AND FILM

The depiction of antipsychotic drugs in entertainment and media has been subject to much discussion for the last few decades. Overall, many works do attempt to show narratives of these medications that coincide with scientifically supported treatment methods. While there is substantial evidence stemming from a biological basis that the use of medication is an effective treatment method for certain conditions such as schizophrenia, empathetic understanding and a loving relationship that might be depicted in works of media have not been proven to cure such illnesses (3). Incorrect notions regarding antipsychotic drugs may be propagated through inaccurate representations of the medications themselves as well as the disorders they target (3).

With the propagation of visual media consumption, television and film have become a way for mental illness and its treatment to be depicted on screen to an audience with vivid detail. A renowned work of 20th century cinema concerning this topic is the 2001 film A Beautiful Mind. The movie is based on the story of mathematician John Forbes Nash Jr. and chronicles his battle with schizophrenia over the course of his life (4).

Initially, antipsychotic drugs are shown in the film as a better treatment option compared to the harsh experimental methods when treatment was still being developed at the time to which John, played by Russel Crowe, is seen subjected to(4). The medication he is prescribed appears as a way for patients to be able to lead normal lives. However, his pills seem to be effective almost immediately, as if patients can get back to their lives within a short period of time (4). The treatment journey of the patients seems as if a brief stay at the hospital and the prescription of medicine is sufficient for a return to regular life. In fact, the real John continued to struggle with his condition for several decades and experienced extended periods of being unable to do his work (4).

The additional conditions accompanying the use of antipsychotic drugs become more evident later on in the film as John attempts to resume his daily routine and research in mathematics (4). Unfortunately, he finds that the medication he is obligated to take to manage his disability is hindering his ability to think and any progress in his academic work (4). The conflicting nature of the drug's influence on his mind and body leaves John with a dilemma. It is apparent that the medication may not provide a complete, cure-all solution to the concerned illness, and this remains a key motivation for continued research into this area.

Patient non-compliance in medication consumption resulting from undesirable side effects is exemplified as John decides to stop taking the drugs in order to think better. As he enters relapse, he becomes delusional and his animated hallucinations cause him to unintentionally do harm to his infant child and wife (4). The message of the film here, according to ABC News, may be that the medication remains a crucial component to the treatment process despite not being a complete solution (4).

An intricate representation of antipsychotic drugs in television is the American "Showtime" thriller series *Homeland* that aired from 2011 to 2020 (5). The show introduces high-level CIA operative Carrie Mathison (Clare Danes) who specializes in post-9/11 anti-terrorism work located in the Middle East (5). Diagnosed with bipolar disorder, Carrie treats her condition first with lithium, later on with antipsychotics like clozapine and Seroquel, and eventually Electroconvulsive "Shock" Therapy (ECT) (5).

The prominence of medication in Carrie's character is shown in her disarrayed medicine cabinet, a prop that might itself be seen as a primary character. Her illness appears to the audience to be inextricably connected with the medications that she chooses to (or not to) intake, and accurate portrayal as seen from a psychopharmacological perspective (5). The first episode "Pilot" features Carrie nervously taking what looks like a bottle of aspirin out of her medicine cabinet without any revelation of her mental health issues. The drugs themselves are shown to be the central indicator of Carrie's illness rather than any explicit symptoms or evidence suggesting she has bipolar disorder (5).

*Homeland* proceeds to depict the relationship with antipsychotics as a substantial indication of underlying mental illness. Max (Maury Sterling), Carrie's co-worker, accidentally discovers that her pills are oblong in shape and green-ish in colour, exposing them as obviously non-aspirin (5). Another co-worker, Virgil (David Marciano) finds after some investigation that the pills are the atypical antipsychotic clozapine (5). Only then does Virgil conclude that Carrie might have a severe mental health condition (5). Later on, Carrie's medicine cabinet makes another two appearances, meaning her medication is explicitly pointed out a total of five times in a single episode (5). In its beginnings, the show portrays medication as a point of inferral regarding the patient's disease for those who are unaware of its presence.

The secrecy surrounding patient consumption of prescribed antipsychotic medication is explored in Carrie's concealment of her pills in relation to her mutuals. While she has adjusted her behaviour well enough to avoid suspicion of her bipolar disorder from the CIA for over 10 years, her pills are also under the cover of an aspirin bottle (5). Even when they are finally discovered, the presence of her illness is only detected through deduction, leading to her being exposed as bipolar.

Though being a part of treatment, the medication faces resistance as well when *Homeland* portrays the act of regularly keeping up with pills as an often laborious responsibility. Maggie, Carrie's sister and unofficial shrink, constantly repeats to her she must remember to take her meds (5). Maggie furthermore patronizes her sister for refusing to seek additional proper treatment such as psychosocial therapy (5). As Carrie exhibits signs of resentment towards her pills, she is also in a way avoiding other therapeutic methods that may be available (5).

Another integral facet to antipsychotics exemplified in *Homeland* is the potential of drug abuse. In the seventh season of the series, Carrie begins to spiral into mania and starts herself on sedating antipsychotic Seroquel (quetiapine fumarate) in order to relax her over-occupied brain (5). However, similar to John Nash from A Beautiful Mind, she wants to maintain a state of mental acuteness in the face of the medications' side effects (4,5). She decides to also take cognitive enhancers such as prescription Adderall (amphetamine/dextroamphetamine), methylphenidate (generic Ritalin) as well as Strattera (atomoxetine) that she purchases from a street-dealer's car (5). Carrie toggles with her arsenal of pills in an attempt to find an equilibrium point of mental keenness (5), exhibiting the potential for antipsychotics to be used irresponsibly on their own and in synergy with other medication.

What's more, it appears that Carrie tries to exploit her mental condition more than manage it. She toggles her use of drugs that treat and intentionally worsen her illness, a neverending neurochemical tug-of-war, with the hope of ultimately benefiting herself from the condition itself (5). Antipsychotic medication is shown as not only a method for treating mental health illness, but a potential way to manipulate a condition within the patient.

### ANTIPSYCHOTIC MEDICATIONS ACROSS CULTURES

The perception of certain medications under cultural and societal influences has a substantial impact on its use in medical practice. The effects can even extend past explanations of the medication's biological function (6).

Examples of sociocultural factors are compliance behavior, social networking in using medicines, beliefs and expectations surrounding the illness, the treatment's mechanisms of action, propensity to placebo-related effects, and use of herbal and strategies from traditional medicines (6).

A patient's willingness to accept prescribed medication is related to variability in drug tolerance and metabolism across cultures, their previous experiences and their current beliefs and perceptions regarding the type of drug (6).

It would appear that attitudes towards Western medicine vary across the globe. Studies from the late 20th century found that patients from East Asian commonly thought that Western medicines were more potent and had greater adverse effects than herbal or traditional methods (6). Though data relating to such topics might be regarded as subjective experiences in contrast to direct pharmacological impact, this remains clinically significant (6). Cases of negative subjective response have been found to be connected to patient non-compliance and poor therapeutic results for medications such as neuroleptics and antidepressants (6). Subjective experiences of medication (as opposed to direct pharmacological effects) are clinically important and should not be dismissed or regarded as non-specific (6). Furthermore, undesirable side effects may perpetuate established biases and deepened unfavorable attitudes in cultural contexts where the opinion of Western medicines is already low (6).

One commonly used self-report scale to gauge societal opinion of neuroleptic treatment in research and clinical settings is the Drug Attitude Inventory (DAI) (6). For this method, items are sorted into seven categories such as subjective negative and subjective positive (6).

The Medication Attitude Scale (MAS) is a more recently developed method that was featured in a 2008 study of cultural factors related to psychotropic medications (6). It was intended as a self-rating scale to quantify attitudes towards psychotropic drugs, including those that were culturally based (6).

Building upon the pre-established DAI, this novel scale integrated the assessment of attitudes as well as perception of drug effects in patients from varying cultures. The method involves 25 individual items in the form of short direct statements that were scored using a four-point scale with labels "completely true," "mostly true," "mostly false," and "completely false" to measure an item's relevance to the patient (6). Thus, views regarding medications could be evaluated based on the degree of prevalence for the individual being surveyed, rather than just a confirmation response one might obtain using a true-or-false system (6). The study cast light upon the dual presence of both positive and negative attitudes held by patients since there is a subjective weighting of apparent benefits and apparent harms that factors into an individual's acceptance of medication.

The participants of the study were broadly identified as Asian and Caucasian, with 51 and 36 patients respectively (6). Of these patients, those who met DSM-IV criteria for chronic schizophrenia were in one group was given clozapine while the other group fulfilling criteria for major depressive disorder was treated with sertraline (6). It was found that patients identifying as Asian expressed less positive attitudes for medications in comparison to Caucasian patients, even when they experienced fewer side effects (6). There was no evident significant difference in total MAS scores in relation to other variables of age, gender or diagnosis (6). It should be noted that while these results may reflect differences due to cultural values regarding medications and their expected effects, other factors such as experience of previous side effects and illness course may have also influenced the attitudes.

Following the perpetual development of human perspectives, it is possible that the current portrayal of antipsychotic medications in modern culture and society will be subject to change in the future. As the relationships between patient and physician, and patient and medication evolve, the need for further research will persist in order to foster the responsible and effective usage of such drugs.

# CHAPTER 11
## CHALLENGES AND FUTURE DIRECTIONS

### Arnavi Patel

#### INTRODUCTION

Antipsychotic medications have been used for many years in the treatment of psychosis. However, they are not without challenges. Although antipsychotic medications have been overall effective, there are still some improvements that need to be made. In this chapter, some challenges of antipsychotic medications, and possible solutions will be explored. These challenges include the lack of knowledge regarding length of treatment, resistance to treatment, the failure to reduce negative symptoms, and the inability of antipsychotics to modify the disorder long term.

#### OPTIMAL LENGTH

Treatments of psychosis with the use of antipsychotics are often meant to decrease symptoms and prevent relapse and hospitalization. However, the length of maintaining treatment once a patient has recovered from an acute episode is unknown (1). Treatments are often continued long term to prevent relapses, however the medications can cause side effects, such as weight gain, which can shorten lifespan (1). A review by Taylor & Ng (2012) examined studies which tested the effects of long-lasting antipsychotic injections. Three studies that were included in this review found patients had significant weight gain during the study (2). The first study showed a mean increase in body mass index (BMI) of 4.8 kg/m2 in the first 12 months of treatment (2). The second study showed a BMI increase of 0.6 kg/m2 from the beginning of the study to the end (2). Furthermore,the third study showed an increase of 0.007 kg/m2 (2). Moreover, antipsychotic medications have failed to be effective for the past two to three years in randomized double blind controlled studies (1).

Some naturalistic studies do show the effectiveness of antipsychotic medications past the two to three year mark, however these studies have limitations to them (1).

To determine an optimal length for antipsychotic treatment, it is crucial for longer and larger randomized controlled studies to take place (1). These studies may be hard to coordinate due to the extensive amount of time and resources needed. However, with the cooperation of different organizations such as international institutions, pharmacies, and governments these studies may be more feasible (1). Larger studies will require larger sample sizes which can account for participants who drop out, and allow for follow up of the patients (1). Oftentimes, some participants may drop out of studies for a multitude of reasons. However, participants dropping out of studies can affect the overall results quite substantially. Larger sample sizes allow for participants to drop out of studies without severely affecting the overall results. With more accurate results, it may be easier to identify an optimal time for the length of treatment. Furthermore, follow up with participants is crucial since antipsychotic medications have the goal of reducing the risk of relapse in the long term (1). Gathering more data from follow up studies may help to better understand the possible side effects which may occur (1). This will also help determine an optimal length of treatment and possible solutions for adverse side effects.

## TREATMENT RESISTANCE

Some patients who experience episodes of psychosis may experience it differently from others. Consequently, patients may not respond to treatments in the same way. Therefore, another one of the many challenges that come with antipsychotic medications is identifying which patients need these medications (1). Approximately ⅓ of patients have treatment resistant illness and 15% show resistance to treatment from the onset of psychosis (1). There are many hypotheses as to why patients may resist treatment. Two of interest are the dopamine supersensitivity hypothesis and genetic variants (3). The dopamine supersensitivity hypothesis states that continuously blocking the dopamine D2 receptor (DRD2) may cause changes to the release of dopamine (See Figure 3)(3). These changes may lead to symptoms that are no longer able to be treated by available medication (3). Furthermore,this can lead to the need to increase doses of medication and continuous treatment (3). Therefore, the longer the treatments are carried on for, the greater the resistance to treatment will be (3). The second hypothesis, the genetic variants, states that changes in certain genes are linked to treatment resistance (3). One of the genetic variants that has been linked to treatment resistant psychosis is polymorphisms in the dopamine transporter (DAT-40) and serotonin transporter (SERT-VNTR) (3). Studies show a base pair variable number of tandem repeats in the dopamine transporter and a polymorphism at intron 2 of the serotonin transporter contributed to development of treatment resistance (3). Furthermore,polymorphisms in DRD2 also affected risks of developing treatment resistance (3). Lastly, two gene sets have also been implicated in development of treatment resistant psychosis (3). Genes relevant to N-methyl-D-aspartate (NDMA) and GRIN2a gene sets are often associated with antipsychotic treatment targets (3). However, variants in these genes have been found which are linked to treatment resistance (3).

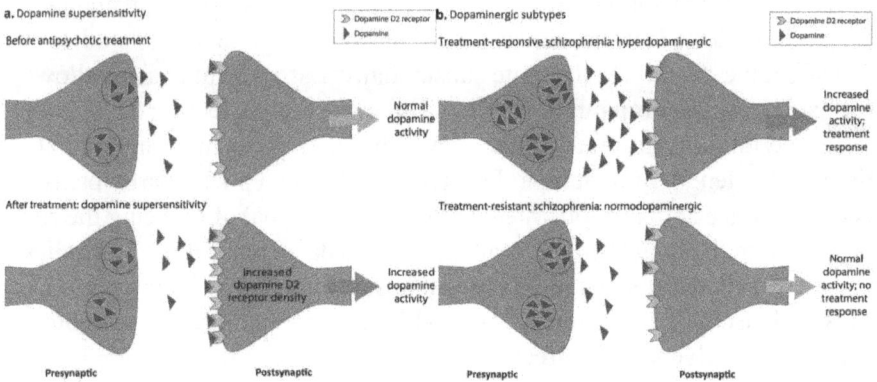

Figure 3: Dopamine Supersensitivity Hypothesis (3)

Furthermore,studies also show development of negative symptoms of psychosis may be linked to treatment resistance in children (4). One study examined the relationships between treatment failure in children and early onset psychosis. They found children with negative symptoms are less likely to continue medication due to insufficient results and adverse effects (4). The study also found children with negative symptoms have lower rates of medicine adherence (4). Medicine adherence refers to the patient's ability to follow medical advice (2). The study also found 30% of children with negative symptoms developed multiple treatment failure (4). This is twice as much as patients without negative symptoms (4). In order to accurately identify patients who may be resistant to antipsychotics, it is crucial to identify biomarkers linked to treatment resistance (1). Hypotheses regarding why patients develop treatment resistance is an essential first step in the right direction. For example, genetic variants can possibly be used to identify biomarkers to assess how well patients will respond to antipsychotic treatments. Further research is needed to assess biomarkers for treatment resistant psychosis.

## LACK OF REDUCTION IN NEGATIVE SYMPTOMS

The third challenge that has been associated with antipsychotic medications is the lack of reduction in negative and cognitive symptoms (1). Antipsychotics have been effective in treating positive symptoms of psychosis, however cognitive symptoms are associated with poor functional outcome (1). Some dopamine agonists have also been linked to causing secondary negative and cognitive symptoms (1). For reference, primary negative symptoms are defined as symptoms that occur without the influence of other medications or other symptoms (5). Whereas secondary negative symptoms, such as anxiety, depression, delusions and hallucinations, are symptoms that are the results of medications or other symptoms (5). Studies with risperidone and haloperidol have shown these antipsychotics may increase negative symptoms, especially avolition and apathy (5).

Studies which measure the effects of antipsychotics on positive and negative symptoms have also failed to clearly show the effects of antipsychotics on negative symptoms (5). Oftentimes studies compare the effects of antipsychotics to a placebo or other antipsychotics, however few studies have evaluated the direct effects of antipsychotics on the primary negative effects of psychosis (5). Therefore, in the available literature it is often difficult to discern whether the treatments affect primary negative symptoms or secondary ones (5). In studies which evaluate the effect of antipsychotics on secondary negative symptoms, amisulpride, clozapine, olanzapine, and risperidone have shown a small to medium effect size (d = 0.54) (5). However, studies with clozapine fail to show effects on primary negative symptoms, despite it being considered one of the strongest antipsychotic medications available (5). Furthermore,amisulpride, haloperidol, olanzapine, quetiapine, risperidone, and ziprasidone have all been shown to treat negative symptoms better than a placebo (5). However, the reductions in negative symptoms occur at the same time as reductions in positive symptoms, during the early stages of treatment (5). Therefore these medications are not considered to cause improvements of primary negative symptoms (5).

For future studies of antipsychotic medications, it is essential to evaluate the reductions in primary negative symptoms. It is also imperative to measure the development of secondary negative symptoms for the duration of treatment. With more research into negative symptoms of psychosis and better methods to treat them, the inability to treat negative symptoms may be overcome.

The fourth challenge that has been identified with antipsychotics is lack of modification of the disorder for long term recovery (1). Current medications act on the post synapses, however, psychosis is linked to pre synaptic striatal dopamine dysfunction (1). Medications have failed to address the underlying dysfunctions of dopamine, which exist long term post treatment (1). The failure to address these underlying causes may also be linked to patient relapses (1). Furthermore,the dopamine supersensitivity hypothesis may also explain the existence of dysfunctions post treatment. As mentioned earlier, the dopamine supersensitivity hypothesis states that continuously blocking the dopamine receptor causes changes to the release of dopamine to the point where medications no longer have the same effect (3). Current medications may continue to cause changes in dopamine rather than solving the underlying issues which can lead to relapse in the long term (3).

A study reviewed the current literature regarding antipsychotic medications and long term effects (6). This study found that patients using antipsychotic medications are at a greater risk of relapse than those who do not (6). Antipsychotic maintenance treatment may help to reduce the risk of relapse after two years, however most studies do not follow up with patients past two years (6). Therefore, the reliance of antipsychotic maintenance treatment to reduce the risk of relapse post treatment is not based on evidence (6). Furthermore,patients who were not prescribed antipsychotic medications showed significantly fewer psychotic symptoms and a better clinical outcome that those who were prescribed antipsychotic medication (6). Comparisons between antipsychotic maintenance treatment and reduction of antipsychotic use also showed that the reduction of use had a greater impact on patients in the long term (6). After 18 months of treatment, those who reduce their use of antipsychotic medications experienced a relapse rate twice as high as those in the antipsychotic maintenance treatment (6). However after seven years, those who reduced their use of antipsychotics showed twice the recovery rate (6). The results from this study indicate antipsychotic medications may have detrimental effects in the long term (6). It is important to address the underlying issues of psychosis to prevent detrimental long term effects of antipsychotic medications.

A possible solution to this challenge is the use of long-acting injections (LAIs). These were developed for patients who have low medicine adherence to oral antipsychotics (2). Long-acting injections of antipsychotics have been tested to decrease rates of relapse and hospitalization in the first episode and early schizophrenia (2). These studies found that relapse rates for patients using LAIs were significantly lower than those using a placebo (2). One study shows 41% of participants who were using a placebo experienced a relapse after the treatment ended, however no patients who were using LAIs experienced a relapse (2). Furthermore,another study shows patients using LAIs were 59% less likely to discontinue treatment than patients who were using oral antipsychotics (2). Patients using LAIs were also at a significantly lower risk of hospitalization than patients using oral antipsychotics (2). Yet another study shows 78% of patients using LAIs showed a meaningful clinical response and only 4 relapsed (2). The adherence for medication was significantly higher for LAIs than oral antipsychotics at one and two years of treatment (2). Long-acting injections are a promising solution to achieving long term recovery from psychosis (2).

Further studies should focus on the use of long-acting injections beyond a specific population. These alternatives to oral medications may be beneficial in treating underlying causes of psychosis and preventing relapse. Other possible treatments which focus on modifying the disorder should also be sought out. Current medications provide treatment while patients are still using antipsychotics. However it is important to research medications which address the underlying causes.

## FUTURE DIRECTIONS

Research shows trends in the prescription of antipsychotic medications are increasing. One study shows a growing increase in antipsychotic medication prescriptions in Pakistan (7). The use of antipsychotics is 4.3 times greater than previous years, which indicates more people are being treated for psychosis than ever before (7).The use of antipsychotics will only grow. However, to ensure patients receive the best care it is important to address the challenges that are currently present. Aside from the four challenges that have been discussed in this chapter there are many more that exist. With further advances in antipsychotic medications, new challenges and limitations may emerge. Therefore it is important to continue research in this field.

## CONCLUSION

As discussed in this chapter, there are many solutions that can help overcome the challenges antipsychotic medications currently face. To summarize, research should focus on identifying an optimal length of treatment by conducting larger studies, identifying biomarkers to assess how patients may respond to treatment, improving antipsychotic medications to address the lack of treatment of negative and cognitive symptoms, and improving antipsychotic medications to address underlying causes of psychosis (1-6). Future research into these areas of antipsychotic medications may help to find solutions to these current challenges.

# REFERENCES

## CHAPTER 1

1. Shen WW. A history of antipsychotic drug development. Comprehensive Psychiatry. 1999;40(6):407–14.
2. Cunningham OD, Johnstone EC. The development of antipsychotic drugs. Brain Neurosci Adv. 2018;2:2398212818817498. Published 2018 Dec 5. doi:10.1177/2398212818817498
3. Muench J, Hamer AM. Adverse effects of antipsychotic medications. Am Fam Physician. 2010;81(5):617-622.

## CHAPTER 2

1. Antipsychotic Medication [Internet]. CAMH. The Centre for Addiction and Mental Health; [cited 2021 May 14]. Available from: https://www.camh.ca/en/health-info/mental-illness-and-addiction-index/antipsychotic-medication
2. Patel, K. R., Cherian, J., Gohil, K., & Atkinson, D. (2014). Schizophrenia: overview and treatment options. P & T : a peer-reviewed journal for formulary management, 39(9), 638–645.
3. NHS Choices. NHS; [cited 2021 May 14]. Available from: https://www.nhs.uk/mental-health/conditions/bipolar-disorder/treatment/
4. Tampi, R. R., Tampi, D. J., Balachandran, S., & Srinivasan, S. (2016). Antipsychotic use in dementia: a systematic review of benefits and risks from meta-analyses. Therapeutic advances in chronic disease, 7(5), 229–245. https://doi.org/10.1177/2040622316658463
5. Wang, P., & Si, T. (2013). Use of antipsychotics in the treatment of depressive disorders. Shanghai archives of psychiatry, 25(3), 134–140. https://doi.org/10.3969/j.issn.1002-0829.2013.03.002
6. 1. Mood Stabilizing Medication [Internet]. CAMH.ca. 2021 [cited 14 May 2021]. Available from: https://www.camh.ca/en/health-info/mental-illness-and-addiction-index/mood-stabilizing-medication
7. Pies R. (2009). Should psychiatrists use atypical antipsychotics to treat nonpsychotic anxiety?. Psychiatry (Edgmont (Pa. : Township)), 6(6), 29–37.

8. Aguilar EJ, Siris SG. Do antipsychotic drugs influence suicidal behavior in schizophrenia? Psychopharmacol Bull. 2007;40(3):128-42. PMID: 18007574.

9. Budman CL. The role of atypical antipsychotics for treatment of Tourette's syndrome: an overview. Drugs. 2014 Jul;74(11):1177-93. doi: 10.1007/s40265-014-0254-0. PMID: 25034359.

10. Thamby, A., & Jaisoorya, T. S. (2019). Antipsychotic augmentation in the treatment of obsessive-compulsive disorder. Indian journal of psychiatry, 61(Suppl 1), S51–S57. https://doi.org/10.4103/psychiatry.IndianJPsychiatry_519_18

11. Stein M, Roy Byrne P, Friedman M. Pharmacotherapy for posttraumatic stress disorder in adults [Internet]. UpToDate. UpToDate; [cited 2021May14]. Available from: https://www.uptodate.com/contents/pharmacotherapy-for-posttraumatic-stress-disorder-in-adults#H5614726

12. Wasylyshen, A., & Williams, A. M. (2016). Second-generation antipsychotic use in borderline personality disorder: What are we targeting?. The mental health clinician, 6(2), 82–88. https://doi.org/10.9740/mhc.2016.03.82

13. Sultan RS, Wang S, Crystal S, Olfson M. Antipsychotic Treatment Among Youths With Attention-Deficit/Hyperactivity Disorder. JAMA Netw Open. 2019;2(7):e197850. doi:10.1001/jamanetworkopen.2019.7850

14. Thompson W, Quay TAW, Rojas-Fernandez C, Farrell B, Bjerre LM. Atypical antipsychotics for insomnia: a systematic review. Sleep Med. 2016 Jun;22:13-17. doi: 10.1016/j.sleep.2016.04.003. Epub 2016 May 11. PMID: 27544830.

15. Posey, D. J., Stigler, K. A., Erickson, C. A., & McDougle, C. J. (2008). Antipsychotics in the treatment of autism. The Journal of clinical investigation, 118(1), 6–14. https://doi.org/10.1172/JCI32483

16. McQuire, C., Hassiotis, A., Harrison, B. et al. Pharmacological interventions for challenging behaviour in children with intellectual disabilities: a systematic review and meta-analysis. BMC Psychiatry 15, 303 (2015). https://doi.org/10.1186/s12888-015-0688-2

CHAPTER 3

1. Canada H. Government of Canada [Internet]. Canada.ca. / Gouvernement du Canada; 2020 [cited 2021May11]. Available from: https://www.canada.ca/en/health-canada/services/drugs-health-products/medeffect-canada/safety-reviews/atypical-antipsychotics-assessing-potential-risk-drug-reaction-eosinophilia-systemic-symptoms.htm

2. Goldburg J. Psychosis: Definition, Symptoms, Causes, Diagnosis, Treatment [Internet]. WebMD. WebMD; 2019 [cited 2021May11]. Available from: https://www.webmd.com/schizophrenia/guide/what-is-psychosis#:~:

text=Psychosis%20is%20a%20condition%20that,or%20trauma%20can%20 cause%20it.

3.  Mental Health I. Drug Approval Process [Internet]. Institute for Advancements in Mental Health - I am mental health. 2021 [cited 2021May12]. Available from: https://www.iamentalhealth.ca/Find-Support/Medication-Resource-Centre/drug-approval-process

4.  Canada H. Government of Canada [Internet]. Canada.ca. / Gouvernement du Canada; 2015 [cited 2021May14]. Available from: https://www.canada. ca/en/health-canada/services/drugs-health-products/drug-products/fact-sheets/drugs-reviewed-canada.html

5.  Canada SP. The Drug Review and Approval Process in Canada - An eGuide: SPharm - Canada's Drug Regulatory Experts [Internet]. SPharm. SPharm - Canada's Drug Regulatory Experts; 2021 [cited 2021May14]. Available from: https://spharm-inc.com/the-drug-review-and-approval-process-in-canada-an-eguide/

6.  Seroquel Medication Guide [Internet]. Access Data . AstraZeneca ; 2011 [cited 2021May14]. Available from: https://www.accessdata.fda.gov/drugsatfda_docs/label/2011/020639s055MG.pdf

7.  Schulman JS. In Vivo vs. In Vitro: What Does It All Mean? [Internet]. Healthline. 2019 [cited 2021May14]. Available from: https://www.healthline.com/health/in-vivo-vs-in-vitro#takeaway

8.  Stroup TS, Leiberman JA, Hamer RM, Alves WM. Clinical trials for antipsychotic drugs: design conventions, dilemmas and innovations [Internet]. Nature reviews. Drug discovery. U.S. National Library of Medicine; 2006 [cited 2021May14]. Available from: https://pubmed.ncbi.nlm.nih. gov/16518380/

9.  Harrow M, Jobe TH, Faull RN, Yang J. A 20-Year multi-followup longitudinal study assessing whether antipsychotic medications contribute to work functioning in schizophrenia [Internet]. Psychiatry research. U.S. National Library of Medicine; 2017 [cited 2021May15]. Available from: https://www.ncbi.nlm.nih.gov/pmc/articles/PMC5661946/

10.  Symptoms - Schizophrenia [Internet]. NHS Choices. NHS; 2019 [cited 2021May15]. Available from: https://www.nhs.uk/mental-health/conditions/ schizophrenia/symptoms/

11.  Foebel A, Ballokova A, Wellens NIH, Fialova D, Milisen K, Liperoti R, et al. A retrospective, longitudinal study of factors associated with new antipsychotic medication use among recently admitted long-term care residents [Internet]. BMC Geriatrics. BioMed Central; 2015 [cited 2021May16]. Available from: https://bmcgeriatr.biomedcentral.com/articles/10.1186/ s12877-015-0127-8

1. Mental Health Medications. Natl Inst Ment Heal. 2021;1–13.

2. Meltzer HY, Gadaleta E. Contrasting Typical and Atypical Antipsychotic Drugs. Focus (Madison). 2021;19(1):3–13.

3. Meltzer HY. Update on typical and atypical antipsychotic drugs. Annu Rev Med. 2013;64:393–406.

4. Kudo S, Ishizaki T. Pharmacokinetics of haloperidol. An update. Clin Pharmacokinet. 1999;37(6):435–56.

5. Tyler MW, Zaldivar-Diez J, Haggarty SJ. Classics in Chemical Neuroscience: Haloperidol. ACS Chem Neurosci. 2017;8(3):444–53.

6. Cooper P. Drugs for schizophrenia. Midwife Health Visit. 1974;10(5):129.

7. Shen YZ, Peng K, Zhang J, Meng XW, Ji FH. Effects of Haloperidol on Delirium in Adult Patients: A Systematic Review and Meta-Analysis. Med Princ Pract. 2018;27(3):250–9.

8. Chipps J. Haloperidol Discontinuation for People with Schizophrenia. Issues Ment Health Nurs. 2020;(4):1–2.

9. Boyd-Kimball D, Gonczy K, Lewis B, Mason T, Siliko N, Wolfe J. Classics in Chemical Neuroscience: Chlorpromazine. ACS Chem Neurosci. 2019;10(1):79–88.

10. Adams CE, Awad GA, Rathbone J, Thornley B, Soares-Weiser K. Chlorpromazine versus placebo for schizophrenia. Cochrane Database Syst Rev. 2014;2014(1).

11. Hartung B, Sampson S, Leucht S. Perphenazine for schizophrenia. Cochrane Database Syst Rev. 2015;2015(3).

12. Cooper P. Perphenazine versus low-potency first-generation antipsychotic drugs for schizophrenia. Midwife Health Visit. 1974;10(5):129.

13. Del Fabro L, Delvecchio G, D'Agostino A, Brambilla P. Effects of olanzapine during cognitive and emotional processing in schizophrenia: A review of functional magnetic resonance imaging findings. Hum Psychopharmacol. 2019;34(3).

14. Khorassani F, Saad M. Intravenous Olanzapine for the Management of Agitation: Review of the Literature. Ann Pharmacother. 2019;53(8):853–9.

15. Casey AB, Canal CE. Classics in Chemical Neuroscience: Aripiprazole. Physiol Behav. 2014;63(8):1–18.

16. Prommer E. Aripiprazole: A New Option in Delirium. Am J Hosp Palliat Med. 2017;34(2):180–5.

1. Antipsychotics - What you need to know. [Internet]. rethink.org. [cited 16 May 2021]. Available from: https://www.rethink.org/advice-and-information/living-with-mental-illness/medications/antipsychotics/

2. NIMH » What is Psychosis? [Internet]. Nimh.nih.gov. [cited 16 May 2021]. Available from: https://www.nimh.nih.gov/health/topics/schizophrenia/raise/what-is-psychosis#:~:text=During a period of psychosis,do not see or hear)

3. Anquil Tablets - Summary of Product Characteristics (SmPC) - (emc) [Internet]. Medicines.org.uk. [cited 16 May 2021]. Available from: https://www.medicines.org.uk/emc/product/6580/smpc#gref

4. Chlorpromazine: Uses, Interactions, Mechanism of Action | DrugBank Online [Internet]. Go.drugbank.com. [cited 16 May 2021]. Available from: https://go.drugbank.com/drugs/DB00477

5. Chlorpromazine 100mg Tablets - Summary of Product Characteristics (SmPC) - (emc) [Internet]. Medicines.org.uk. [cited 16 May 2021]. Available from: https://www.medicines.org.uk/emc/product/3476/smpc

6. Flupentixol: Uses, Interactions, Mechanism of Action | DrugBank Online [Internet]. Go.drugbank.com. [cited 16 May 2021]. Available from: https://go.drugbank.com/drugs/DB00875

7. Depixol Tablets 3mg - Summary of Product Characteristics (SmPC) - (emc) [Internet]. Medicines.org.uk. [cited 16 May 2021]. Available from: https://www.medicines.org.uk/emc/product/997/smpc

8. Berman B. Neuroleptic Malignant Syndrome. The Neurohospitalist [Internet]. 2011 [cited 16 May 2021];1(1):41-47. Available from: https://www.ncbi.nlm.nih.gov/pmc/articles/PMC3726098/#:~:text=Neuroleptic%20malignant%20syndrome%20(NMS)%20is,muscle%20rigidity%2C%20and%20autonomic%20dysfunction

9. Haloperidol: Uses, Interactions, Mechanism of Action | DrugBank Online [Internet]. Go.drugbank.com. [cited 16 May 2021]. Available from: https://go.drugbank.com/drugs/DB00502

10. Haldol 2mg/ml oral solution - Summary of Product Characteristics (SmPC) - (emc) [Internet]. Medicines.org.uk. [cited 16 May 2021]. Available from: https://www.medicines.org.uk/emc/product/180/smpc

11. Methotrimeprazine: Uses, Interactions, Mechanism of Action | Drug-Bank Online [Internet]. Go.drugbank.com. [cited 16 May 2021]. Available from: https://go.drugbank.com/drugs/DB01403

12. Levomepromazine Hydrochloride 25mg/ml Solution for Injection - Summary of Product Characteristics (SmPC) - (emc) [Internet]. Medicines.org.uk. [cited 16 May 2021]. Available from: https://www.medicines.org.uk/emc/product/3014/smpc

13. Periciazine: Uses, Interactions, Mechanism of Action | DrugBank

Online [Internet]. Go.drugbank.com. [cited 16 May 2021]. Available from: https://go.drugbank.com/drugs/DB01608

14. Pericyazine 10mg Tablets - Summary of Product Characteristics (SmPC) - (emc) [Internet]. Medicines.org.uk. [cited 16 May 2021]. Available from: https://www.medicines.org.uk/emc/product/3969/smpc

15. Perphenazine: Uses, Interactions, Mechanism of Action | DrugBank Online [Internet]. Go.drugbank.com. [cited 16 May 2021]. Available from: https://go.drugbank.com/drugs/DB00850

16. Pimozide: Uses, Interactions, Mechanism of Action | DrugBank Online [Internet]. Go.drugbank.com. [cited 16 May 2021]. Available from: https://go.drugbank.com/drugs/DB01100

17. Orap 4 mg tablets - Summary of Product Characteristics (SmPC) - (emc) [Internet]. Medicines.org.uk. [cited 16 May 2021]. Available from: https://www.medicines.org.uk/emc/product/6911

18. Promazine: Uses, Interactions, Mechanism of Action | DrugBank Online [Internet]. Go.drugbank.com. [cited 16 May 2021]. Available from: https://go.drugbank.com/drugs/DB00420

19. Promazine Hydrochloride 25mg/5ml Oral Syrup - Summary of Product Characteristics (SmPC) - (emc) [Internet]. Medicines.org.uk. [cited 16 May 2021]. Available from: https://www.medicines.org.uk/emc/product/6697/smpc

20. Sulpiride: Uses, Interactions, Mechanism of Action | DrugBank Online [Internet]. Go.drugbank.com. [cited 16 May 2021]. Available from: https://go.drugbank.com/drugs/DB00391

21. Sulpiride 200mg Tablets - Summary of Product Characteristics (SmPC) - (emc) [Internet]. Medicines.org.uk. [cited 16 May 2021]. Available from: https://www.medicines.org.uk/emc/product/2430/smpc#

22. Zuclopenthixol: Uses, Interactions, Mechanism of Action | DrugBank Online [Internet]. Go.drugbank.com. [cited 16 May 2021]. Available from: https://go.drugbank.com/drugs/DB01624

23. Clopixol 10 mg film-coated tablets - Summary of Product Characteristics (SmPC) - (emc) [Internet]. Medicines.org.uk. [cited 17 May 2021]. Available from: https://www.medicines.org.uk/emc/product/11789/smpc

24. Amisulpride 100 mg Tablets - Summary of Product Characteristics (SmPC) - (emc) [Internet]. Medicines.org.uk. [cited 17 May 2021]. Available from: https://www.medicines.org.uk/emc/product/2726/smpc

25. Amisulpride: Uses, Interactions, Mechanism of Action | DrugBank Online [Internet]. Go.drugbank.com. [cited 17 May 2021]. Available from: https://go.drugbank.com/drugs/DB06288

26. Aripiprazole: Uses, Interactions, Mechanism of Action | DrugBank Online [Internet]. Go.drugbank.com. [cited 17 May 2021]. Available from: https://go.drugbank.com/drugs/DB01238

27. Abilify 1 mg/mL Oral Solution - Summary of Product Characteristics (SmPC) - (emc) [Internet]. Medicines.org.uk. [cited 17 May 2021]. Avail-

able from: https://www.medicines.org.uk/emc/product/8954/smpc#CLINI-CAL_PRECAUTIONS

28. Clozapine: Uses, Interactions, Mechanism of Action | DrugBank Online [Internet]. Go.drugbank.com. [cited 17 May 2021]. Available from: https://go.drugbank.com/drugs/DB00363

29. Clozaril 100 mg Tablets - Summary of Product Characteristics (SmPC) - (emc) [Internet]. Medicines.org.uk. [cited 17 May 2021]. Available from: https://www.medicines.org.uk/emc/product/10290/smpc#CLINICAL_PRE-CAUTIONS

30. Risperidone: Uses, Interactions, Mechanism of Action | DrugBank Online [Internet]. Go.drugbank.com. [cited 17 May 2021]. Available from: https://go.drugbank.com/drugs/DB00734

31. Risperdal 0.5mg Film-Coated Tablets - Summary of Product Characteristics (SmPC) - (emc) [Internet]. Medicines.org.uk. [cited 17 May 2021]. Available from: https://www.medicines.org.uk/emc/product/6856/smpc

32. Olanzapine 10 mg Film-coated Tablets - Summary of Product Characteristics (SmPC) - (emc) [Internet]. Medicines.org.uk. [cited 17 May 2021]. Available from: https://www.medicines.org.uk/emc/product/6082/smpc

33. Olanzapine: Uses, Interactions, Mechanism of Action | DrugBank Online [Internet]. Go.drugbank.com. [cited 17 May 2021]. Available from: https://go.drugbank.com/drugs/DB00334

34. Quetiapine: Uses, Interactions, Mechanism of Action | DrugBank Online [Internet]. Go.drugbank.com. [cited 17 May 2021]. Available from: https://go.drugbank.com/drugs/DB01224

## CHAPTER 6

1. Steigman AJ, Vallbona C. Chlorpromazine, a useful antiemetic in pediatric practice. The Journal of Pediatrics. 1955;46(3):296–7.

2. Sadove MS. Chlorpromazine and Narcotics In The Management of Pain of Malignant Lesions. Journal of the American Medical Association. 1954;155(7):626.

3. Stroup TS, Gray N. Management of common adverse effects of antipsychotic medications. World Psychiatry. 2018;17(3):341–56.

4. Relling MV, Mulhern RK, Fairclough D, Baker D, Pul C-H. Chlorpromazine with and without lorazepam as antiemetic therapy in children receiving uniform chemotherapy. The Journal of Pediatrics. 1993;123(5):811–6.

5. Srivastava M, Brito-Dellan N, Davis MP, Leach M, Lagman R. Olanzapine as an Antiemetic in Refractory Nausea and Vomiting in Advanced Cancer. Journal of Pain and Symptom Management. 2003;25(6):578–82.

6. Robertson MM, Trimble MR. Major tranquilisers used as antidepressants. Journal of Affective Disorders. 1982;4(3):173–93.

7. Philip NS, Carpenter LL, Tyrka AR, Price LH. Augmentation of Antide-

pressants with Atypical Antipsychotics: A Review of the Current Literature. Journal of Psychiatric Practice. 2008;14(1):34–44.

8. Nelson JC, Papakostas GI. Atypical Antipsychotic Augmentation in Major Depressive Disorder: A Meta-Analysis of Placebo-Controlled Randomized Trials. FOCUS. 2010;8(4):570–82.

9. Shafiq S, Pringsheim T. Using antipsychotics for behavioral problems in children. Expert Opinion on Pharmacotherapy. 2018;19(13):1475–88.

10. Lamberti M, Siracusano R, Italiano D, Alosi N, Cucinotta F, Di Rosa G, et al. Head-to-Head Comparison of Aripiprazole and Risperidone in the Treatment of ADHD Symptoms in Children with Autistic Spectrum Disorder and ADHD: A Pilot, Open-Label, Randomized Controlled Study. Pediatric Drugs. 2016;18(4):319–29.

11. Miller L, Riddle MA, Pruitt D, Zachik A, dosReis S. Antipsychotic Treatment Patterns and Aggressive Behavior Among Adolescents in Residential Facilities. The Journal of Behavioral Health Services & Research. 2013;40(1):97–110.

12. Schur SB, Sikich L, Findling RL, Malone RP, Crismon ML, Derivan A, et al. Treatment Recommendations for the Use of Antipsychotics for Aggressive Youth (TRAAY), Part I: A Review. FOCUS. 2004;2(4):596–607.

13. Weisman H, Qureshi IA, Leckman JF, Scahill L, Bloch MH. Systematic review: Pharmacological treatment of tic disorders – Efficacy of antipsychotic and alpha-2 adrenergic agonist agents. Neuroscience & Biobehavioral Reviews. 2013;37(6):1162–71.

14. Huys D, Huys D. Update on the role of antipsychotics in the treatment of Tourette syndrome. Neuropsychiatric Disease and Treatment. 2012;:95.

15. Hershenberg R, Gros DF, Brawman-Mintzer O. Role of Atypical Antipsychotics in the Treatment of Generalized Anxiety Disorder. CNS Drugs. 2014;28(6):519–33.

16. Weber SR, Wehr AM, Duchemin A-M. Prevalence of antipsychotic prescriptions among patients with anxiety disorders treated in inpatient and outpatient psychiatric settings. Journal of Affective Disorders. 2016;191:292–9.

17. Schneider LS, Dagerman K, Insel PS. Efficacy and Adverse Effects of Atypical Antipsychotics for Dementia: Meta-analysis of Randomized, Placebo-Controlled Trials. The American Journal of Geriatric Psychiatry. 2006;14(3):191–210.

18. Kales HC, Kim HM, Zivin K, Valenstein M, Seyfried LS, Chiang C, et al. Risk of Mortality Among Individual Antipsychotics in Patients With Dementia. American Journal of Psychiatry. 2012;169(1):71–9.

19. Barnes TR, Banerjee S, Collins N, Treloar A, McIntyre SM, Paton C. Antipsychotics in dementia: prevalence and quality of antipsychotic drug prescribing in UK mental health services. British Journal of Psychiatry. 2012;201(3):221–6.

20. Thompson W, Quay T, Rojas-Fernandez C, Farrell B, Bjerre L. Atypical antipsychotics for insomnia: a systematic review. Sleep Medicine. 2016;22:13–7.

21. Bullard DE. Metoclopramide: Pharmacology and clinical application. Journal of Oral and Maxillofacial Surgery. 1983;41(11):753.

22. Lee A, Kuo B. Metoclopramide in the treatment of diabetic gastroparesis. Expert Review of Endocrinology & Metabolism. 2010;5(5):653–62.

### CHAPTER 7

1. Chokhawala K, Stevens L. Antipsychotic Medications. [Updated 2020 Oct 23]. In: StatPearls [Internet]. Treasure Island (FL): StatPearls Publishing; 2021 Jan-. Available from: https://www.ncbi.nlm.nih.gov/books/NBK519503/

2. Dopamine and T cells: dopamine receptors and potent effects on T cells, dopamine production in T cells, and abnormalities in the dopaminergic system in T cells in autoimmune, neurological and psychiatric diseases. Acta Physiol., 216 (1) (2016), pp. 42-89

3. Shen WW. A history of antipsychotic drug development. Compr Psychiatry. 1999 Nov-Dec;40(6):407-14. doi: 10.1016/s0010-440x(99)90082-2. PMID: 10579370.

4. Seeman P. Atypical antipsychotics: mechanism of action. Can J Psychiatry. 2002 Feb;47(1):27-38. PMID: 11873706.

5. Stahl SM. "Hit-and-Run" actions at dopamine receptors, part 2: Illustrating fast dissociation from dopamine receptors that typifies atypical antipsychotics. J Clin Psychiatry. 2001 Oct;62(10):747-8. doi: 10.4088/jcp.v62n1001. PMID: 11816862.

6. Swartz MS, Stroup TS, McEvoy JP, Davis SM, Rosenheck RA, Keefe RS, Hsiao JK, Lieberman JA. What CATIE found: results from the schizophrenia trial. Psychiatr Serv. 2008 May;59(5):500-6. doi: 10.1176/ps.2008.59.5.500. PMID: 18451005; PMCID: PMC5033643.

7. Simpson GM. Atypical antipsychotics and the burden of disease. Am J Manag Care. 2005 Sep;11(8 Suppl):S235-41. PMID: 16180961.

### CHAPTER 8

1. Catherine R. Glenn, Joseph C. Franklin & Matthew K. Nock (2015) Evidence-Based Psychosocial Treatments for Self-Injurious Thoughts and Behaviors in Youth, Journal of Clinical Child & Adolescent Psychology, 44:1, 1-29, DOI: 10.1080/15374416.2014.945211

2. Dilip V. Jeste, Jeanne E. Maglione, Treating Older Adults With Schizophrenia: Challenges and Opportunities, Schizophrenia Bulletin, Volume 39,

Issue 5, September 2013, Pages 966–968, https://doi-org.proxy.bib.uottawa.ca/10.1093/schbul/sbt043

3. Robert S. Kern, Shirley M. Glynn, William P. Horan, Stephen R. Marder, Psychosocial Treatments to Promote Functional Recovery in Schizophrenia, Schizophrenia Bulletin, Volume 35, Issue 2, March 2009, Pages 347–361, https://doi-org.proxy.bib.uottawa.ca/10.1093/schbul/sbn177

### CHAPTER 9

1. Antipsychotics - What you need to know. [Internet]. Antipsychotics. 2021 [cited 16 May 2021]. Available from: https://www.rethink.org/advice-and-information/living-with-mental-illness/medications/antipsychotics/

2. Bhandari S. Antipsychotic Medication for Bipolar Disorder [Internet]. WebMD. 2020 [cited 16 May 2021]. Available from: https://www.webmd.com/bipolar-disorder/guide/antipsychotic-medication

3. Haddad P, Sharma S. [Internet]. Adverse Effects of Atypical Antipsychotics. 2012 [cited 14 May 2021]. Available from: https://link.springer.com/article/10.2165/00023210-200721110-00004

4. Mental Health Medications [Internet]. Nimh.nih.gov. 2016 [cited 16 May 2021]. Available from: https://www.nimh.nih.gov/health/topics/mental-health-medications/

5. Schaffer AL, Zoega H, Tran DT, Buckley NA, Pearson S, Havard A. Trajectories of antipsychotic use before and during pregnancy and associated maternal and birth characteristics. Australian & New Zealand Journal of Psychiatry. 2019 Dec;53(12):1208-21

6. What Are Bipolar Disorders? [Internet]. Psychiatry.org. 2021 [cited 12 May 2021]. Available from: https://www.psychiatry.org/patients-families/bipolar-disorders/what-are-bipolar-disorders#:~:text=Bipolar%20disorder%20is%20a%20brain,to%20weeks%2C%20called%20mood%20episode

### CHAPTER 10

1. Munce SE, Robertson EK, Sansom SN, Stewart DE. Who Is Portrayed in Psychotropic Drug Advertisements? Journal of Nervous & Mental Disease [Internet]. 2004Apr1 [cited 2021May10];192(4):284–8. Available from: https://europepmc.org/article/med/15060402

2. Hansen FJ, Osborne D. Portrayal of Women and Elderly Patients in Psychotropic Drug Advertisements. Women & Therapy [Internet]. 1995Jul [cited 2021May11];16(1):129–41. Available from: https://www.tandfonline.com/doi/abs/10.1300/J015v16n01_08

3. Owen PR. Portrayals of Schizophrenia by Entertainment Media: A Content Analysis of Contemporary Movies. Psychiatric Services [Internet].

2012Jul [cited 2021May10];63(7):655–9. Available from: https://ps.psychia-tryonline.org/doi/pdf/10.1176/appi.ps.201100371

4. A Beautiful Mind: Analyzing How Schizophrenia is Portrayed in Movies versus Reality [Internet]. Disability in Media Review Blog. The Ohio State University; [cited 2021May10]. Available from: https://u.osu.edu/kovacev-ich.9/sample-page/

5. Bennett R. The Psychopharmacological Thriller: Representations of Psychotropic Pills in American Popular Culture. Literature and Medicine [Internet]. 2019 [cited 2021May10];37(1):166–95. Available from: https://muse.jhu.edu/article/7308286.

6. Ng CH, Klimidis S. Cultural factors and the use of psychotropic medica-tions. Ethno-psychopharmacology [Internet]. 2008 [cited 2021May11];:123–34. Available from: https://www.cambridge.org/core/books/ethnopsycho-pharmacology/cultural-factors-and-the-use-of-psychotropic-medications/CB29E87F83474687B94CD083A938FE00

## CHAPTER 11

1. Howes OH, Kaar SJ. Antipsychotic drugs: challenges and future direc-tions. World Psychiatry. 2018 Jun;17(2):170–1.

2. Taylor M, Ng KYB. Should long-acting (depot) antipsychotics be used in early schizophrenia? A systematic review. The Australian and New Zealand journal of psychiatry. 2012 Dec 3;47.

3. Potkin SG, Kane JM, Correll CU, Lindenmayer J-P, Agid O, Marder SR, et al. The neurobiology of treatment-resistant schizophrenia: paths to anti-psychotic resistance and a roadmap for future research. npj Schizophrenia. 2020 Jan 7;6(1):1–10.

4. Downs J, Dean H, Lechler S, Sears N, Patel R, Shetty H, et al. Negative Symptoms in Early-Onset Psychosis and Their Association With Antipsy-chotic Treatment Failure. Schizophrenia Bulletin. 2019 Jan 1;45(1):69–79.

5. Aleman A, Lincoln TM, Bruggeman R, Melle I, Arends J, Arango C, et al. Treatment of negative symptoms: Where do we stand, and where do we go? Schizophrenia Research. 2017;186(Complete):55–62.

6. Murray RM, Quattrone D, Natesan S, van Os J, Nordentoft M, Howes O, et al. Should psychiatrists be more cautious about the long-term prophylactic use of antipsychotics? Br J Psychiatry. 2016 Nov;209(5):361–5.

7. Mahmood S, Hussain S, ur Rehman T, Barbui C, Kurdi AB, Godman B. Trends in the prescribing of antipsychotic medicines in Pakistan: im-plications for the future. Current Medical Research and Opinion. 2019 Jan 2;35(1):51–61.

www.ingramcontent.com/pod-product-compliance
Lightning Source LLC
Chambersburg PA
CBHW021829190326
41518CB00007B/791